THIN KIDS

THIN

THE PROVEN, HEALTHY, SENSIBLE PROGRAM

Mindy Cohen M.A. and

BEAUFORT BOOKS

KIDS

FOR CHILDREN WHO WANT TO

- Lose Weight
- Improve Their Self-Image
- Deal With Food Problems at Home and at School
- Choose the Right Fast Foods
- Cope with Food "Pushers"
- Relax With Techniques to Relieve Stress
- Start an Exercise Program That Works
- Stay Fat-Free Forever

Louis Abramson
With Ruth Winter

PUBLISHERS NEW YORK

Copyright © 1985 by Mindy Cohen, Louis Abramson, and Ruth Winter.

All rights reserved. No part of this publication may be reproduced or transmitted in any form or by any means, electronic or mechanical, including photocopy, recording, or any information storage and retrieval system now known or to be invented, without permission in writing from the publisher, except by a reviewer who wishes to quote brief passages in connection with a review written for inclusion in a magazine, newspaper, or broadcast.

Library of Congress Cataloging in Publication Data

Cohen, Mindy.
   Thin kids.

   1. Obesity in children. 2. Reducing diets.
   3. Children—Nutrition. I. Abramson, Louis.
II. Winter, Ruth,
1930– . III. Title.
RJ399.C6A23   1985   613.2'5'088054   84-24492
ISBN-0-8253-0276-5
ISBN 0-8253-0277-3 (pbk.)

Published in the [United States] by Beaufort Books Publishers, New York.

Designer: Christine Swirmoff / Libra Graphics, Inc.

Printed in the U.S.A.   First Edition

10 9 8 7 6 5 4 3 2

To Philip with love

CONTENTS

FOREWORD by Lester L. Coleman, M.D.   **ix**
INTRODUCTION: How Thin Kids Began   **xiii**

PART I: GETTING STARTED

CHAPTER I: Talking It Over with Your Child   **3**
CHAPTER II: How to Begin   **11**
CHAPTER III: Fighting Temptation and Finding Rewards   **19**

PART II: THE PROGRAM

CHAPTER IV: At Home and at School—The Challenges   **29**
CHAPTER V: Temptation Times—Holidays, Parties, Vacations, Outings   **34**
CHAPTER VI: Love with Calories—Dealing with Food Pushers   **43**
CHAPTER VII: Fighting Fat with Fun and Games   **50**
CHAPTER VIII: The Thin Kids Stress Relievers   **79**

PART III: FACING FACTS ABOUT FOOD

CHAPTER IX: Nutrition: What Every Thin Kid Should Know   **85**
CHAPTER X: Quiz: How Much Have You Learned About Food?   **92**
CHAPTER XI: Hints and Suggestions from Mindy, Lou, and Some Thin Kids   **98**

PART IV: THE THIN KIDS FOOD PLAN

CHAPTER XII: *Ten Weeks of Thin Kids Menus*   **105**
CHAPTER XIII: *Thin Kids Recipe Section*   **181**
CHAPTER XIV: *Fat Free Forever*   **203**
APPENDIX: *Food Groups*   **205**

FOREWORD

No single concept or theory can possibly untangle the myriad ramifications that exist in the understanding and treatment of obesity.

Almost all people, scientists and laity alike, who depart from the fundamental truth of the causes of obesity are certain that they have within their grasp the complete answers to the total problem that now exists in epidemic form.

Sincere but often unrealistic approaches to this disorder of modern civilization can confuse rather than clarify the issues. To be overweight is to have excessive burdensome weight. Obesity suggests corpulence and the accumulation of excessive fat. Like caution and cowardice, one is the trade name for the other. Numerous technical and scientific descriptions have been made of the content of fat cells in the body. These minute chemical and physiological studies are far too confusing for the untrained, unscientific mind.

Obesity is a disease of magnitude that demands the cooperative efforts of physicians, psychologists, scientists, and social observers if it is to be prevented, controlled, and cured. Included in their observations are all the physical, chemical, nutritional, emotional, ethnic, social metabolic, familial, and psychological implications of overweight and obesity.

With so many variables in the equation of obesity, no single answer exists. Yet we cannot be deflected from our search if the child, the adolescent, and the adult are to be spared the hazardous threat of obesity to health and life.

The social stigmatizing effects of obesity deprive persons of all ages of many of the opportunities, privileges, and happy experiences to which they might be heir. The obese person in our society bears that social burden because of changes in physical attractiveness. Prejudice and even ridicule are irrational reactions to many obese people. Obesity, therefore, is an albatross that must be eliminated early in life. For it is undeniable that the fat infant becomes the fat child and then the fat adolescent and finally the fat adult.

Since there are so many familial, social, genetic, and hormonal factors involved in obesity, every avenue must be explored to interrupt this progression. Only then can the individual be spared the frustrations, the personal dissatisfactions, the depression, the anxiety, and the interference with social progression.

In order to attain the ultimate objectives of good health, physical and emotional, a remarkable program has recently been devised. An innovative Thin Kids Program™ has been created by Mindy Cohen and Louis Abramson. Highly trained in the subtleties of nutrition, exercise, and psychological attitudes, Mindy Cohen and Louis Abramson have already proven the efficacy of their program. Under their supervision, children debilitated by the burden of obesity are being taught to reorient their total patterns of eating and exercise. The weight loss and psychological guidance give children an excellent insight into their problems and, by cooperative efforts, achieve the solutions.

What is particularly exciting about the Thin Kids Program is the mutual support that emerges among parents, siblings, and Thin Kids registrants. Spurred by this intrafamilial support, a weight reduction program emerges, one that motivates other members of the family to attain similar health objectives.

It must be emphasized that bad diets, pharmacological treatments, and psychotherapeutic approaches continue to evolve. Some flourish while others end in precipitous failure.

I am most enthusiastic about the fundamental concepts incorporated in the Thin Kids program. It is a significant multifaceted approach to the obesity problem, the solution of which offers the greatest assurance that the child, armed with

FOREWORD

a new image, will attain adolescence and adulthood as a happier and more productive member of society.

Lester L. Coleman, M. D. Attending Surgeon, Otolaryngology, Manhattan Eye, Ear and Throat Hospital; Clinical Professor, Otolaryngology, Albert Einstein College of Medicine, New York City; Syndicated Medical Columnist, King Features Syndicate, New York City; Past President, American Academy of Psychosomatic Medicine.

INTRODUCTION: HOW THIN KIDS BEGAN

When I was eight years old, I, Mindy, used to watch *I Dream of Jeannie* on TV. Jeannie was a genie who could make wishes come true. I had one wish. I wanted to be thin!

By the time I was thirteen, my parents had taken me to dozens of specialists from endocrinologists to medical school pediatricians. I had undergone a series of injections. I had become addicted to water pills that interfered with my normal metabolism. I had been to adult diet groups, at least half a dozen. Besides feeling out of place at the diet groups, I could not relate to the others. How could they understand what it is like to be in the school cafeteria or understand the problems I had after school? They were more concerned about what to do when their spouses were home.

I tried over-the-counter diet aids. The products that are supposed to take your appetite away gave me an appetite. I would eat my way through a whole box. I read books and tried carbohydrate-free diets. I would lose a few pounds and then regain them.

At thirteen, when adolescents are supposed to be blossoming, I was ballooning. I was five foot three and weighed 145 pounds.

My parents spent a lot of money in a desperate attempt to help me. They knew how unhappy I was.

I would have given anything to be picked for a team at

school. I was always the one who remained. The gym teacher took pity on me and made me the captain. But, no matter how hard I tried, I could never get more than a C in gym.

I, Lou, teach elementary school physical education and I am also certified to teach health and psychology. When I first met Mindy, physical education had failed her. Her lifestyle was typical of the time. Her family had two cars so she was driven everywhere. She took elevators and escalators, never climbing stairs unless there was absolutely no alternative. Mindy attended schools during a period when physical education was geared mainly to give children physical tests and teaching them sports. She was always the last one chosen for a team and she was humiliated when she had to try to climb a rope or sprint or do any sort of gymnastics. As for a bathing suit, she would have rather had her teeth drilled than to appear in one in public.

Lou is absolutely right! I would not get into a bathing suit unless I could cover it up with a big T-shirt. In fact, all of my clothing in my teenaged years was the peasant type, large and shapeless.

The only exercise I got was walking to school, which was less than half a mile from my home. Even at that, I was so sluggish that some mornings I didn't want to get up and go to school because I had to walk there. Any physical activity was just too much of an effort.

When I was thirteen, I was invited to a party, a rare event because I had been left out of most birthday parties and other social events. No one asked me to dance. Finally, one boy did. I knew it was because he felt sorry for me.

I had read something in the "Dear Abby" column about a girl who was fat and unattractive in high school and no one paid any attention to her. Then the boy who had been the most popular in her class meets her ten years later. She is thin and gorgeous and he tries to date her but she will not have anything to do with him because he insulted her in high school. I consoled myself that someday I would be that girl.

I even felt strongly as a youngster that my parents were ashamed of my weight. I thought that they did not accept me for what I was.

INTRODUCTION

I have a very thin sister. This is not uncommon. My mother was also very thin. When I became a school psychologist, I asked my sister, who is older, how she was able to remain thin. She said she would model herself after my mother. She also said that she was always involved in a lot of activities and was able to keep herself thin by being busy. She was very social and met the man who was to be her husband when she was fifteen years old.

I was close to my father who was overweight and loved to eat. When we had pizza, my father would tell me I was looking fat so he could have the last slice. Even though I knew why he said it, the words hurt.

On Saturday nights entertainment for my parents was going out to dinner. Since I was the overweight adolescent with no one to go out with, I would tag along with my parents. My sisters were older and were out on dates.

I have to say my father literally gave his life for food. He lived to eat and when he would get too overweight, he would go on the latest diet. The last one he tried was a popular low carbohydrate diet where you were allowed to eat as much fat as you want. At forty-five-years-old and with an undiagnosed coronary condition, he was eating things like sausage, bacon, and eggs.

When I was fourteen, my father died of a massive coronary. So I was struggling alone with my weight and the problems it caused. By the time I reached twenty, I weighed 160 pounds. I was more desperate than ever. I tried injections. They didn't work. I tried diet pills and went back to the same doctor that I had as a youngster. Again I failed to control my weight.

The turning point in my life in my war against obesity was meeting Lou in college. He was a health and physical education major and a champion fencer, and I was studying psychology. We both had an interest in nutrition. I from the psychological aspect and he from the physical fitness one. He convinced me about the importance of exercise in weight loss and I convinced him of the importance of family interaction and emotions. Based on our studies in college, we both realized that I could have been helped as a child to achieve normal weight and maintain it but that there was no program specifically designed for the special problems of overweight children. I, Mindy, decided to take my masters in psychology and to make my field of study childhood weight problems.

I conducted a research project in a hospital with medical and psychological supervision. The techniques I developed there—based on my own experience as a fat child and upon nutritional and psychological research—were then tested by a large pediatric group in New Jersey. Ten patients were enrolled in an initial test group. The results were good. The children lost eight to ten pounds in ten meetings.

I, Lou, was by then a physical education and health teacher. I joined the second test group and began teaching youngsters about the benefits of exercise and gave them easy ways to be more active.

We found that in the second group, the children's weight loss almost doubled what the first group had lost in the ten weeks. The doctors began referring more and more children. Other pediatricians began requesting the program and school nurses asked to send students. Hospitals requested our program. The reason it was so popular among medical personnel was that they had long seen the great need for such help for overweight youngsters but did not have the time or special methods of giving it. The demand became so great that we had to move from the pediatric groups offices into our own. Within five years our program has spread to five locations in the New York–New Jersey area.

When I, Mindy, did my thesis, I chose nine- to twelve-year-olds because when I was nine that was the first time I was taken to a doctor and failed to lose weight. I know what it is to be a fat child. I've been through it. There are many health reasons that a child should not be overweight but one of the most important of all is that many obese youngsters are unhappy. They are robbed of many of the joys of childhood—the physical and social activities. In our society there is a prejudice against the fat child. Their peers torment them with name calling and teachers and other adults tend to be less tolerant. Some adults believe obese children are lazy and weak-willed. In one classic study, results showed that college admission personnel were more inclined to reject the

CHAPTER 1

TALKING IT OVER WITH YOUR CHILD

Some parents of overweight children are overweight themselves and/or were overweight as children. Some parents of overweight children are thin. We, Mindy Cohen and Lou Abramson, have come into contact with more than a thousand youngsters and their parents through the Thin Kids program. We have found that there is one thing that all the mothers and fathers share in common: They love their children and want them to be healthy and happy!

When your child is hurt emotionally or physically, you feel the pain. Joan Lake, for example, was with her six-year-old daughter, Tina, in a supermarket. They met another mother with a daughter who was in Tina's dancing class.

"You remember her," the child pointed at Tina. "She's the one with the fat legs!"

The youngster's remark brought back all the pain and humiliation of Joan Lake's own childhood.

"When I was in the third grade, I weighed one hundred and ninety pounds," the small blond employee of a fast food chain in New Jersey recalled. "The children used to torment me by calling me Elsie The Cow. I didn't want Tina to go through the same thing."

Tina, a cute, light-brown haired child, was more than twenty percent above the average weight for her age, height, and bone structure.

"Her costume was always the last to be made in dancing school," her mother recalled. "The other girls took a size six but she was a size ten."

Joan and Tina shared their experiences and feelings with others at a Thin Kids session. Each group meets once a week for ten weeks. Youngsters of all ages sit around a semi-circle and their parents sit around the outside. We do not separate the children by age because we have found that the experience of children who have had to deal with obesity in our society gives them a common bond of understanding that crosses the age and social barriers. The older children can really empathize with the younger children and the younger ones really listen to the older ones because they know they have gone through the same thing.

Even parents who have not experienced being overweight themselves can provide valuable insight about the special problems a thin parent faces when trying to help an obese child.

Jennie Kalen, R. N., the mother of nine-year-old Mary, for example, had never been overweight in her life. Blond and beautiful, she looked more like a fashion model than nurse. Mary, at eight, was four feet eight inches tall and weighed 113 pounds. The kids called her fatso and she had trouble running. She was so overweight she was knock-kneed.

"I never blamed her for being fat. I blamed myself," Jennie said. "My husband's a policeman who worked nights and the kids and I ate a lot of fast foods. My other daughter is as thin as a rail but Mary kept getting heavier. As both a nurse and a mother, I realized I had the responsibility for Mary's health and had to do something about her weight. I asked Mary if she wanted to try the Thin Kids program."

Mary did and she explained to us why: "I have a lot of friends but I don't do well at sports. I have trouble fitting into clothes. I don't like the way I look."

Tina, six, on the other hand, was reluctant to go. When her mother finally convinced her to try the program, she sat through the first session without volunteering a word. During a Thin Kids class, there is a lot of free and lively exchange between children and between parents and children. Tina evidently absorbed some of the knowledge and spirit because she did lose two pounds the first week. By the second session she responded when asked. By the third week she was a full participant and eager to come even after she had finished the ten week program.

"It was the first five pounds," Joan Lake said. "When my daughter saw that she could do it, she was an emotionally and physically changed child."

"It was the new clothes," Tina said. "My Mom didn't have to take me to the chubby department anymore."

Both Tina and her mother felt rewarded by the successful loss of weight. That is one of the keys to the success of Thin Kids. We emphasize both the emotional and physical rewards that can be achieved.

Many parents, like Jennie Kalen, feel guilty about their child's obesity. They blame themselves for not being able to control their youngster's food intake. Almost all feel frustrated and not infrequently the dinnertable becomes a battle ground.

Dr. James Kantor, a pediatrician, knows well the battleground of the family dinnertable.

"A lot of people take my advice, but not my son," Dr. Kantor explained. "I tried to control his eating but he'd just keep grabbing food and eating off everyone else's plate. I'd come down at midnight, and he'd be at the refrigerator. One of my colleagues told me about Thin Kids, so I brought Petie to a class. I admit that I felt kind of guilty about being so busy and not paying enough attention to him.

"I found the program is absolutely nutritionally and medically sound. I learned to relax a little more from the other parents and Petie seemed right away to be willing to follow the program because he found the other kids in the class did. I even learned some things myself. I do the shopping with my wife on Saturdays and now we're both very careful about what we select and bring home."

As Dr. Kantor noted, we at Thin Kids emphasize to parents that your child has to feel it is his choice to lose weight, not yours or anyone else's.

Sam, a husky salesman who attended the same meetings that Dr. Kantor did, found that out. He tried to threaten, bribe, and tease his twelve-year-old son, Mike, into losing weight.

"My kid was studying to be a whale," Sam said rather loudly. Sam had a booming voice and entertained the whole group. He was crazy about his son, that was obvious, but he didn't realize how teasing and name calling hurt Mike and made matters worse. Teasing, although well meant, is not the wise approach.

Many overweight youngsters, like Mike, are so sensitive and have been so hurt by their peers' name calling—we all know that kids can be cruel—that it is difficult for a loving parent to even broach the subject of weight loss. How should you begin?

First of all, you have to be supportive and you have to offer concrete, educational advice, as will be shown in this book. You have to work with your child and together target those behaviors that lead to overeating.

In a study of more than two hundred children enrolled in the Thin Kids program, we found a number of interesting statistics. The children in the study ranged from six years to seventeen years; the lightest was sixty-eight pounds and the heaviest 230 pounds. The average age of "becoming overweight" was 6.24 years. In twenty-eight percent of the cases both mother and father were overweight and in ten percent, there were overweight siblings. In only sixteen percent no other family member was overweight.

The clients listed why they believed they were overweight:

NIGHT EATING	33 percent
BINGE EATING	25 percent
SNACKS	85 percent
MEALS	49 percent

The totals add up to more than one hundred percent because the client could select more than one choice as a possible explanation. But results do show that snacking is probably a major cause of obesity in children and the area that needs a lot of attention. In this book we not only give you healthy, low-calorie snacks that children especially like but we also give you the techniques you can use to help your child avoid snacking.

The statistics showed that forty-three percent of our children had started on other diet regimens and failed. One reason we have been so successful with the Thin Kids program—more than eighty percent lose weight and remained thin—is because it is geared especially to the needs of children.

One of the major premises of Thin Kids and perhaps the greatest contributor to the success of our program is that a child feels he or she has control over his or her weight loss program. Your child, of course, needs your help, but you must make your youngster feel in charge.

Bobby is a prime example. He took it very hard when his parents divorced and he and his mother moved in with his grandmother. His grandmother, in an effort to make Bobby happier, did what many Grandmas would do. She gave her grandson all kinds of treats—cookies, cakes, lasagna, pancakes. Bobby just grew heavier and more unhappy. He was withdrawn at school and his marks fell. His mother had no choice but to work and Bobby missed her as well as his father. He was depressed and isolated and used food as solace.

His mother said, "I was exhausted after work but I felt that something had to be done about Bobby. He wasn't having any fun. He hated school. He had no friends. He'd just stay home with my mother and eat. I felt guilty, frustrated, and very upset about my son. I took him to Thin Kids and I think we both got a lot out of it. I found, first of all, that my problems with Bobby weren't unique. I enjoyed the meetings with the other parents and kids."

We saw immediately that Bobby was a very bright boy. We encouraged his mother to allow him to do some of the supermarket shopping and the cooking to give him some control over his life and his diet. He cooked for the family under the careful supervision of his loving grandmother. Bobby was precise and kept track of his weight, and his calorie intake on his home computer. He lost fifty pounds and was a completely different personality. In fact, from a shy boy he turned into a real personality kid. He joined a Scout troop and made new friends. His marks at school improved dramatically.

The improvement in the entire dynamics of Bobby's family is not unusual. By working on obesity, which is really a family problem even if only one child is overweight, the experience benefits everyone.

Thirteen-year-old Theresa and her mother, for example, did not get along. They were constantly fighting. Connie, Theresa's mother, explained it this way:

> My daughter was a very unhappy child and I was a very unhappy Mom. She was really heavy and she drove me crazy. Our household was always in turmoil. If she dressed to go to a party or a function, she would try on everything in the closet, look at herself, and say, "I'm ugly. I'm fat. I hate myself."
>
> Shopping was horrendous. Everything I brought to the dressing room she hated. She would say, "Everything makes me look fat!" Many, many times, we would leave without buying anything.
>
> She had few friends and if she would go to a party, she would be very shy of strangers. Swim parties were definitely out. Kids were cruel. They teased her and called her names. I went to school to talk to the principal. I called mothers to talk to their children and make them stop tormenting Theresa. The unhappier my daughter got, the more she ate and the more we fought. At the time everyone was wearing a certain designer's jeans. I couldn't find a pair to fit Theresa and she wanted them more than anything in the world. I finally bought a pair of the designer's jeans for men and had them cut to fit my daughter.

Connie wrote us a letter weeks after Theresa had completed the Thin Kids program and while the family was on vacation together:

> Thin Kids helped Theresa lose twenty-five pounds and thus far, she has kept it off. She is literally a different child. She has many friends, girls and boys. In fact, she has gone to the other extreme and is quite social. Shopping is a delight but also sometimes goes to an extreme. Everything looks wonderful. She is into having her hair changed and her face made up. I have to say that her marks have dropped somewhat in school. Theresa used to be an all-A student because all she did was study.

Now she has some B's but we think it is well worth it when we see how happy she is.
 The whole family benefited not only from learning how to eat better and using the Thin Kids program, but working together to help Theresa succeed was also satisfying. I just wanted to thank you for helping Theresa achieve weight control and to find happiness and fun in her thirteenth year of life.

We gain tremendous satisfaction from seeing how weight loss, such as Theresa's, can change a child's social life. Connie put it into a letter, but sometimes it is little things that illustrate it. We both remember well Theresa's face, for instance, the evening she came to class and said, "I walked past a neighbor and she called me by my *sister's* name!" (Theresa's sister had always been slim while Theresa had been very overweight.)
 Just take a moment to picture the changes losing weight could make in your child's life.
 All right. You are ready to help but how do you bring up the subject?

(From now on throughout the book we will interchange he and she because obesity affects both genders equally.)

First of all, don't criticize your child about his obesity and don't necessarily point out the health benefits of losing weight. Many kids are turned off if you say something is "fattening" or "good for you." But if you say losing weight will help you "run faster" or "look better" that has more appeal.
 Ask your child what she thinks the benefits of losing weight really are. Your child may or may not say "looking better." Appearance, of course, is important. Tell your child that even though you think she looks great, she will like what she sees in the mirror better if she does lose weight. Tell her she will also feel better. And, although children find it hard to worry about the future, you can discuss the benefits of controlling weight in childhood to avoid the problems of heart disease and diabetes that overweight adults often have.
 You can discuss the social benefits of being of average

weight. People don't call you "fatty" anymore. But you should be very careful about this delicate topic. Emphasize that you are proud of your child and that your love doesn't depend upon how much he or she weighs. If your youngster says that the kids call him "fatty" and other names, you can point out that problem will disappear along with the weight. If she loves sports, emphasize she will be able to participate instead of watching from the sidelines.

Not all overweight children are unhappy. If yours is not, don't force the issue, even though you know, as a parent, it will be better for his health. Accept it until you can sense that your help in the Thin Kids program would be appreciated. If you force your child on a program or argue about it, the food may become a weapon against parental authority.

If your child is willing and eager, then you, as well as your youngster, will have to change some long-time habits. One of the great things about the Thin Kids program is that usually everyone in the family, overweight and thin alike, learns to eat a healthier diet. And an obese parent or sibling can also lose weight along with the participating child.

CHAPTER II

HOW TO BEGIN

Now that you and your child have embarked on the journey together, the first thing you have to do is to sit down and make a folder. It can be a regular manila folder, a loose leaf notebook, or even a used large manila envelope.

Your child should decorate it. Some like to draw on the folder with crayons or marking pens. Others like to cut out pictures from magazines or buy stickers. Teens should make a folder, too, since it creates something tangible with which to work. That folder is going to be filled by the end of ten weeks not only with papers and charts but with successes.

The first sheet in the folder should be your child's weight loss goal. No child is taken into the Thin Kids program without a physician's recommendation about the amount of weight to be lost. Youngsters, unlike adults, are growing. That's one reason unbalanced crash diets that adults often embark upon are unsafe for youngsters. Children need a nutritionally balanced diet to fuel proper growth and development. Furthermore, for each inch of growth, approximately five pounds are added. Thus, if a child remains the same weight but grows two inches, he may not have to lose as much as an adult might under the same circumstances.

We strongly recommend you have your child examined by his physician and have the doctor prescribe the amount of weight loss your child should set as a goal.

Once you have the goal for the ten weeks set, make ten copies of the weekly food charts and ten copies of the weekly activity charts. (See pages 102–105) Your child should put down everything that is eaten each day, including snacks and where and what they were doing while eating. Your child should write down all activities, including walking to school, sports, walking the dog, cleaning the garage—anything that is active.

In later chapters there will be more about the reasons for writing everything down. If, by the way, your child cannot keep track of things herself, then you can do the recording but let your child dictate the information.

Now with a pad and pencil, your child or you should write down the answers to the questionnaires in Chapters II and III. The answers to the first will help you both pinpoint some of the diet pitfalls and the behaviors that need to be changed. It is also a lot of fun to look back at the answers after the program is completed. The answers to the second will suggest rewards and substitute activities, the importance of which will be described in the next chapter.

INSERT QUESTIONNAIRES

1. Why do you want to lose weight?
2. How much time do you spend on homework?
3. Do you have a particular time and place for homework?
4. Do you have any hobbies?
5. Do you enjoy any sport or physical activity?
6. How much TV do you watch?
7. What are your special responsibilities around the house?
8. Please check any of the following that you believe may explain your weight problem:
   Night eating ____ Binge eating ____ Snacks ____ Meals ____
9. Do you often eat more than fifty percent of a day's food after dinner?

HOW TO BEGIN

10. If you have been on any other diet program, please describe the program and the feelings you had about it.
11. Are you or have you ever been active in an exercise program?
12. What time do you usually:
    Get up in the morning? ____ go to school? ____ get home from school? ____ go to bed? ____ eat breakfast? ____ eat lunch ____ eat dinner? ____ have a snack? ____

There are no right or wrong answers to the above questions. When you and your child go over the information elicited, certain patterns should emerge. The following are the reasons for the questions and an explanation of what the answers may signify and the direction your efforts might take.

1. The reasons usually given are like the following. Some kids think it is a physical and emotional way to feel better. Others say that it is a lot of work for the body to carry around the extra weight. Some kids are unhappy with being overweight and feel a lot of pride and self-esteem when they reach the goal of losing a certain amount of weight. Some kids can't make a team because they are overweight. They are embarrassed during gym or games—always being tagged out when they are trying to reach a base in baseball or coming in last in a race or not even being able to make the race because they are winded and out of condition. Another frequent answer concerns being able to fit into regular clothes. Shopping is often an unhappy experience for an obese child and it is a joyful, proud moment when they find they are several sizes smaller than they were and can get into designer jeans or whatever clothes turn them on.

But a word of caution. Don't stress appearance too much in your discussion. You don't want to give your child the impression that you feel bad about the way they look. Let them mention it themselves. When a kid says, "I don't like the way I look;" we usually say, "You look great the way you are but if you want to look different, that's a fine reason for wanting to lose weight." Health, future health problems may be mentioned. There are some young children who already have high blood pressure, joint problems, asthma, or allergies that may be aggravated by excess weight. A frequent reason for wanting to lose weight, of course, is to stop the other children's name calling. Many obese youngsters become targets.

2. The reason for this question is to identify the problem times. Often kids eat because of boredom. If they can be active with an hour or two of homework, that's less time to think about eating.

3. The kitchen is not a good place to do homework. It becomes a stimulus for eating. Seeing the food, seeing other people eat snacks, or smelling the food as it is being prepared makes it difficult for a youngster to resist.

4. Hobbies, again, will keep a child from "boredom eating."

5. A physical sport, of course, will help with fitness and weight problems. But you have to help your child identify an activity he really likes or he won't keep doing it. If you can find a sport she really likes, it will be an added incentive for losing weight.

6. Commercials on TV stimulate eating. Furthermore, believe it or not, your child can get bored watching TV. If he is used to eating a snack while watching TV, he will have to learn to control the stimulus of TV itself. Ask your child for some suggestions on how she could do that. He may come up with a particularly effective one, because he thought it up.

7. Many kids, because they have working mothers or a single parent home, are responsible for cooking the dinner. That makes weight control for them more difficult. If the family menu is highly caloric, perhaps it could be changed to more low calorie recipes with your help. And if the cooking responsibility can be given to another child, who does not have a weight problem, or to some other member of the family, the obese youngster can earn her keep with other chores.

8. Again, this helps a child define problem times and together you can come up with plans to ease through the periods.

9. If your daughter eats most of her food after dinner or

from dinner time on, her body doesn't have time to digest it and work it off. So, you should work together to balance out the meals.

10. Some kids can fall back on experiences and successes of past weight control efforts. If your child has no experience with a diet, then you have to give him a lot more explanation and support and encouragement to get started. If, on the other hand, he has failed on other diet programs, he may believe he cannot do it. You have to convince him that together, you and he can.

11. If they have been active in an exercise program, that's great. If not, see Chapter VII, page 50.

12. The information elicited here will help plan the day to avoid the "danger" times.

All right, now that you have got the folder and pinpointed some of the problem areas, it is time to start making some changes. The first place you should begin is at the supermarket. It is most important to take your child shopping with you because, as we have emphasized before, your child has to feel control and participation in her own Thin Kids program.

In all the following projects encourage your child to participate. As we keep emphasizing, your child must feel in control of her food program.

THE KITCHEN

Reorganize your shelves. Keep the nutritious, low calorie foods at eye level or within the child's reach. Either get rid of the high calorie, non-nutritious foods or put them out of reach and out of sight and, hopefully, out of mind.

If your child had been doing his homework in the kitchen, find another spot in the house. If you have the TV in the kitchen, move it out if possible. Temptation is just too great if you spend time at non-food tasks in the kitchen. You can fill up a cookie jar with raisins or turn it into a penny bank. Each time the child gets through a period without diverting from the program, you can give her a coin to put into the bank.

If your child helps with chores in the kitchen, let her make the salad or set the table. If he is helping with the dishes, let him wash and dry instead of wrapping up the leftovers.

THE SUPERMARKET

Make up a list with your child of the groceries you will need at the supermarket. Skip the aisle with the cookies and candies and go to the produce department instead. Purchase fresh fruits and vegetables when possible so that you can have cut up celery sticks and carrots and cucumbers in the refrigerator if your child wants a snack. The vegetable sticks will stay fresher if you place them in a glass of water. Also have your child's favorite fruits readily available. And buy juices so you and your child can make ice pops; see page 199. Also buy popcorn. If you have an air popper, that's great because the popcorn won't have any extra calories.

Purchase low fat meats such as chicken, turkey, and fish and buy rice crackers, low calorie ice cream products, and low fat milk. Pita bread and thin-sliced breads are always good to have on hand. They have fewer calories than regular bread. There are many low calorie, delicious selections in the modern supermarket. It is a matter of choosing wisely. And remember, if you don't bring the fattening stuff home, there will be no temptation at home to slip off the food plan.

THE DINING TABLE

You may have to change the family's eating habits. Often today members of the family are so busy they don't have time to sit down and have a relaxing meal together. When they do, tension may be pervasive. How much your child eats at the dinnertable may have little to do with the food served. Michael Lewis, M.D., professor of pediatrics and Director of the Institute for the Study of Exceptional Children at Rutgers Medical School, and his colleagues took video tapes of fifty families from a cross section of socio-economic groups consisting of two parents and one to four children. Among their observations were the following.

HOW TO BEGIN

- Eating is one of the least significant things that happens at the dinnertable.
- The amount of learning that is gained through dinnertable discussion seems minimal.
- Fathers talk more to their sons than to their daughters; mothers talk to fathers more than fathers talk to mothers.
- Middle children are often ignored by both parents.
- Despite the fact that more women are working outside the home, it is still the mothers who prepare and serve the meal in most households.
- Dessert is often used as a bribe to get the children to eat other foods.

The Rutgers researchers found that dinner is a time of regimentation. An enormous number of rules are repeated endlessly—"sit still," "chew slowly," "say please," "don't reach," "use your knife."

Dinner time was found to not be a very happy occasion in most households. What's it like in yours? How can you make the meal more nourishing, emotionally as well as physically?

We urge you to arrange it so that you do eat a pleasant dinner meal with your child, especially if you work and are very busy. The dinner meal should be treated as a festive occasion. Allow your child to make or select colorful placemats, for example. He may want to pick some flowers or pretty fall leaves for the table.

Help your child plan meals and snacks each day that are nutritious and calorie controlled. As we keep pointing out, the more in control of his own diet the child feels, the greater the effort he will make to stick to a food plan. Teach your child to read food labels. Even very young children can learn to identify the various sugars, salts, and calories in food.

Give smaller portions on the plate and put the leftovers away before you even serve the meal so that to have a second helping one would really have to make an effort.

Try to avoid having the dieting child clear the table of food since that offers too much of an opportunity to eat "leftovers."

A tried and true recommendation of behavioral psychologists is to use smaller plates and utensils. That makes less seem like more. A pickle fork or chopsticks are fun for children and they slow down eating.

Encourage your child to cut up her food into as tiny pieces as possible and to chew slowly. Make it a game to see how small she can cut the food. All that helps to regulate food intake. If a child eats slower, she will get full faster.

Keep regimentation or instruction at the table to a minimum. You can always make suggestions after the meal is finished. The meal should be as serene as possible.

Set a good example. The eating habits of parents and older siblings greatly influence a child's food behavior.

By now, we know that mothers and fathers should not force children to clean their plates "because people in Africa [or China or somewhere] are starving." Children will not starve at your table, and even if your child gets on a one-food kick, don't fight it. It will pass, unless, of course, it becomes an area of conflict. Then the emotional garbage may remain.

Allow your child to leave the table as soon as he is finished eating. Waiting around while siblings or parents continue to eat is unfair to the child trying to lose weight.

Do not use food as a reward or punishment. There are other incentives for toilet training and good behavior. Withholding a meal or dessert as punishment certainly gives a confusing psychological message to the child. If you help your child separate physical food from "emotional food," you will have accomplished a great deal.

CHAPTER III

FIGHTING TEMPTATIONS AND FINDING REWARDS

For Timmy it was every time a burger commercial came on TV and it seemed that they did every few minutes.

For Martha it was school birthday parties. She tried to take just one bite of the cake and just one piece of candy, but as most of us know, it is very hard to deliver ourselves from temptation.

If you tease, scold, or over-react when your child overeats or eats the wrong thing, you will be hindering rather than helping your youngster's self-control. Guilt, shame, or anger just add to the problem, and sometimes food can make a good weapon if your child wants to rebel. Your child can develop the ability to handle temptations and to neutralize food pushers with the techniques used in our Thin Kids program. Those techniques involve recognizing the stimuli that causes eating behavior, substituting one behavior for another, and reaping rewards.

First of all, let's deal with stimuli. See if this sounds familiar. Every time Timmy cried as an infant, his mother, Jane, would put a bottle in his mouth.

"My book told me to feed him on demand," Jane explained. "Not like my mother fed my sisters and me when we were babies—by the clock."

When Timmy had his inoculations, his own pediatrician

gave him a lollipop to soothe him. During toilet training, his mother rewarded his efforts with cookies and candy treats.

"He has a mind of his own," Jane said. "I don't believe in hitting my kids so when he refused to eat his vegetables or meat, or pick up his toys, I'd take away his dessert. When he was extra good, I'd let him have chocolate fudge ice cream, his favorite."

Coming from a warm, happy, Irish family, there were a lot of holiday celebrations. The dining room table was always heaped with festive food brought by aunts, cousins, and grandmothers.

When Timmy was a baby, his chubby cheeks and large size delighted his relatives who believed he was the very picture of health. After all, great grandfather emigrated to America so that his children wouldn't starve during the great Irish famine. The first generation had a hard time making ends meet, but Timmy's family had a steady income and money to buy as much food as they needed.

In first grade when Timmy's teacher had to get a large desk for him because he didn't fit into any in the classroom his parents laughed and said, "He's sure a big bruiser."

By the time he came to Thin Kids upon the strong recommendation of his pediatrician, nine-year-old Timmy was wearing "small"-sized clothing but from the men's department.

In Timmy's case his physician felt that both his immediate physical and mental health were at risk because of obesity. His blood pressure and cholesterol levels were already elevated. He was suffering skin rashes from the fat folds rubbing against each other and his breathing was compromised because at four foot three he was, according to the standard charts, thirty-eight pounds overweight.

Timmy had his own reasons for coming to Thin Kids.

"I got sick of the kids calling me 'The Goodyear Blimp' and not being able to run," he said. "I had trouble breathing even when I just walked fast across the room. I wanted to have fun like everyone else."

Timmy, who had the largest blue eyes we ever saw and fiery red hair, had the motivation to lose weight but he had to deal with a lot of temptation that our society, which so loves thinness, puts before overweight youngsters.

FIGHTING TEMPTATIONS

"It was the burger commercials that really got me on TV," Timmy explained. "At first I'd try to just close my eyes and cover my ears whenever they came on. Then I figured something out. Every time a commercial came on, I would run around the house. I had my own track. From the living room, through the kitchen, up the stairs, in my bedroom and my brother's and down the stairs again."

That not only delivered Timmy from the temptation of burger commercials but provided him with some physical exercise, which we'll attend to later. Of course, his parents knew when a burger commercial came on, because the house shook as Timmy made his way around his track but his mother and father felt that was a small price to pay.

For Susan, eight, a child who went through the program with Timmy, it was the candy commercials that got to her. As we emphasize in Thin Kids, children have to find substitute behaviors to counteract old eating habits. Susan came up with the idea of jumping rope during every candy commercial. The jump rope not only helped her resist temptation, but again, greatly increased her physical exercise, especially since candy commercials are so common on children's TV programming.

You may have to help your child identify the eating stimuli in her life and to develop substitute behaviors and to find her own personal rewards.

Often parents have to enlist the help of one of the adults with whom a child spends a lot of time, the school teacher. Martha had a big problem at school. At least twice a week a child had a birthday party and cake, ice cream, and candy were brought in. Martha just couldn't resist eating the treats, even though she was thirty pounds overweight. The other kids, as they often do, kept urging their overweight classmate to pig out on the candy and cake.

With Martha's permission—and that is very important because some children do not want anyone to know about their weight loss program, particularly at school—her mother spoke to her teacher about Martha's efforts to resist temptations. From then on the teacher, unobtrusively, sent Martha on errands out of the classroom while birthday party treats were being served.

Temptation, as we have pointed out, involves stimuli.

Go through the following questions and answers that identify stmuli, resistance, and reward. Even the younger children in the Thin Kids program grasp the concepts quite easily.

WHAT IS BEHAVIOR? *Any way we act is behavior.*

WHAT IS A STIMULUS? *Something that makes us act. It is a signal that makes us act such as a school bell or the telephone ringing or a burger commercial or a birthday cake.*

WHAT IS A RESPONSE? *Any answer by word or act. Everything we do is a response. We may get in line when the bell rings. That is a response to the stimulus (the bell ringing). Timmy got up and ran around the room when the burger commercial came on. He could have eaten a burger. Either would have been a response to the burger commercial.*

WHAT IS A REINFORCER? *A reinforcer is like a reward or a trophy. A reward, trophy, or prize are examples of positive (+) reinforcers because they add to the chances that you will behave the same way you did to earn the reward, trophy, or prize.*

There are also negative (−) reinforcers. Like in arithmetic, when you see the minus (−) sign, you subtract. Negative reinforcers subtract or take away something. When you eat and your hunger or upset feelings go away, that is a negative reinforcer.

When a behavior is reinforced, it will happen more often in the future. If you turn on the TV and it is broken, how many times will you keep turning it on? Wanting to see TV is the reinforcement for turning on the set, but if the set doesn't work, you won't keep trying to turn it on. Behavior needs to be reinforced a number of times before it is learned.

One of the best techniques in weight control, is substituting a behavior for the behavior that involves overeating or eating fattening foods. The following are some examples of substituting behaviors. Try to identify with your child—

FIGHTING TEMPTATIONS

and they may be obvious on the food and activity sheets—the problem times and help your child come up with some good substitute behaviors.

Present Behaviors	**Behavior Changes**
1. Eating candy while riding	Sing along with the radio
2. Eating while watching TV	Painting while watching TV
3. Feeling hungry at 4:00	Going for a walk at 4:00
4. Eating when you're upset	Talking when you're upset
5. Not eating at the kitchen table	Eating only at the kitchen table
6. _____	_____
7. _____	_____
8. _____	_____

POSITIVE REINFORCEMENT OR REWARDS

The biggest rewards your child will receive is losing weight and looking better, feeling better about himself or herself, and improving his or her health. It is also important to reward (reinforce) the behavior changing effort. This will help your child practice the newly learned behaviors.

The following questionnaire is designed to help you and your youngster identify the rewards that would help reinforce your child's determination to control food intake. Select the appropriate reward for a specific goal—say one week of sticking to the program or the loss of two pounds. The more Number 4's your child checks, the easier it will be to find pleasurable activities that will serve as incentives and reinforcements for behavior changes. However, you can use several activities in column Number 2 to add together and make a more powerful incentive for the child who is less enthusiastic and may be more difficult to reward.

Reward and Reinforcement Questionnaire

	Don't like (0)	Like (2)	Like a lot (4)

SHOPPING ACTIVITIES
    Books
    Clothes
    Computers
    Food
    Other

HOBBIES
    Music
    Toys
    Sporting goods
    Video games

WORKING WITH COMPUTERS
    Programming
    Games
    TV
    Movies

SOCIAL ACTIVITIES
    Talking on the phone
    Visiting friends
    Visiting relatives
    Watching people
    Family discussions
    Helping in the classroom,
        at home, in the community
    Scouting

GAMES
    Video games
    Chess
    Checkers
    Jigsaw puzzles
    Other board games

FIGHTING TEMPTATIONS

	Don't like (0)	Like (2)	Like a lot (4)

CRAFTS
Crayoning
Painting or painting by number
Ceramics
Crocheting
Knitting
Rug hooking
Models
Cutting and paste
Collecting stamps, sports cards, coins, etc.
Other

PETS
Bird
Cat
Dog
Fish
Other

PHYSICAL ACTIVITIES
Boating (paddle, rowing, canoeing)
Boxing, wrestling, and team sports
Hiking
Fishing
Running
Other

READING
Books
Magazines
Comics
Other

MUSICAL ENJOYMENT
Playing an instrument
Listening to classical, folk, rock music, jazz, etc.
Other

(You also may want to list the things you like to do best, list what you want to do with your parents, list what you want to do with your friends and use these as rewards.)

Some kids like many different things and find it easy to please themselves. Some children need extra reinforcement from the outside, which might include buying certain things. A reward in our society that always works well is money. You may give a child a coin for every day or meal he stays on the program. You may also offer a dollar a pound. It may be materialistic but it is a very effective incentive. After you and your child have discussed the above, add up the points and select the greatest reward or rewards and write them down. Putting the objective down on paper reinforces determination. When a reward is received after a behavior change, it strengthens or reinforces the behavior so that the next time it needs to be done, it will be easier. Determine when your child will attain that reward. For example, after "one week" on the program or "after losing three pounds."

A word of caution. Make sure the goal is appropriate to a weight loss program. One father wanted to reward his daughter with an ice cream sundae. Another gave his son a video game. In both instances the rewards, while desired by the children, were booby traps. In the first instance, of course, the sundae is loaded with calories and it reinforces the idea that food is a reward and an emotional balm. [In the second case the boy sat in front of the set all day instead of being active.] A football or a tennis racket would have been a better choice.

A reward that involves both you and your child is more desirable. For example a trip to the museum or the zoo—both involve learning and walking—or even window shopping at a mall or sightseeing exercise the mind, the body, and family bonds. And remember, one of the biggest rewards you can give your youngster is a loving hug. It has no calories.

PART 2
THE PROGRAM

CHAPTER IV

AT HOME AND AT SCHOOL— THE CHALLENGES

Pam, a shy thirteen-year-old, not only had the problem of being overweight, but she also had to adjust to a new school, a difficult experience for a brand-new teenager who had spent her childhood in another part of the country.

Pam's father, a professor, has always been as thin as a rail. Her mother on the other hand had tried every radical diet ever publicized but had little success in losing weight and keeping it off. She, too, was very overweight. She brought Pam to Thin Kids because she felt her daughter would have an easier adjustment to the new school if she were of normal weight.

First of all, we discussed with Pam whether or not she wanted her teachers or friends to know that she was on a food program. Some children are absolutely against anyone knowing. They feel that it would add to the teasing and make their school lives more difficult. In fact, this is why other attempts at bringing weight loss classes into the school have not met with much success. The children did not want to be singled out to participate.

On the other hand, schools can be very cooperative. In Pam's case she said she did not want anyone to know. She lost twenty-five pounds while in Thin Kids. The warmth and camaraderie she found at Thin Kids helped her to have a better picture of herself. She blossomed into a lovely young lady and the last we heard from her she was enjoying her new school and doing well.

Lester, an eleven-year-old boy who started the program the same time Pam did, had no objection to his teacher knowing but did not want his classmates to be aware of his efforts.

Lester's teacher was most cooperative. She sent him on errands when there were class parties and, even more important, gave him special jobs to do that helped his self-esteem. As he lost weight, both his teacher and the principal praised him and urged him on.

One major challenge that Pam and Lester and other children trying to lose weight face is the school cafeteria. Starchy and fatty foods are laid before a child in a too tempting display. A child can learn to resist temptation and select salads and lean meats and fruits when possible. However, we suggest that whenever possible it is far easier for a child to brown bag her own lunch. It may take a bit of doing on your part to make sure that lunch is not too different from what the other children have and that your child really likes the content. If not, the lunch will most likely be traded or dropped in the garbage can.

You will want to make sure that there are at least two or three ounces of protein, a fruit, and a starch in the bag. See Chapter XII for brown bag lunch suggestions for school.

You should try to include a treat in the bag. It can be popcorn, a small toy, a game to play with a friend, or a book to read while other children are still eating. It can be as simple as including a pencil in the brown bag so the child can play ticktacktoe with a friend.

CLASS PARTIES

The second greatest challenge in schools is the class party. For the younger grades it is the constant birthday parties and for the teenagers it is the outings and after school gatherings.

AT HOME AND AT SCHOOL

If your child is one who does not mind your contacting the teacher about the food plan, then we urge you to do so not only for your child's sake but for all children present and future in the class. There is no reason why non-fattening, healthy food and drink cannot be offered in place of the sugared punch and candy. See the recipe for Cranberry Cooler on page 187, for example. In addition or in place of the traditional cake, there can be ice cream cake or tropical fruit salad à la mode.

If it is important to him to participate in the party, your child can eat a small piece of cake and leave the icing on the plate. She can cut down on other calories for dinner. But stress this for *special occasions only*. He can drink water in the party cup instead of soda or punch. Instead of sitting at the desk and being tempted, you and your child should brainstorm together to come up with other things to do such as reading a book or playing a board game or doing a puzzle. Often there are children who will eat some food or eat it quickly and then go off to play. Encourage your child to go off and play with those who have finished eating.

If your child finds it really hard to resist all the sugared treats, the teacher could unobtrusively send your child on errands during the eating portion of the party. Pre-planning and rehearsing will make things easier. (See Chapter VI.)

While one of the worst things about being an overweight child is the cruel teasing of other youngsters, not all children are mean. Your child may have some very good friends who could be helpful in aiding his effort to stick to the food plan. Once they are aware of what your child should and should not eat, they can reinforce your youngster's determination and avoid eating fattening foods in front of him.

AFTER SCHOOL AT A FRIEND'S HOUSE

Most children like a snack after school. If your child goes to a friend's house and the friend or the mother offers something not on the food plan—such as brownies, ice cream, or soda, how can your child resist the temptation?

Lester, for example, learned to ask for a piece of fruit or

a glass of water. If there was no fruit, he just said, "I'm not hungry."

Pam usually managed to go home first, eat one of her healthy snacks, and then meet her friends. Other children find it is easier to say, "I'll wait outside for you or in the rec room," while their friends eat their after school snack.

AFTER SCHOOL AT HOME

Have good after school snacks available. You can have raisins, low calorie yogurt, low calorie ice cream pops, broth, V-8 Juice or tomato juice, frozen fruit juicepops, frozen juice ice cubes, salad, and vegetables raw or cooked with a cottage cheese dip. See recipes on page 200–201.

If after school is a challenge time identified by your child, then together you should set up a schedule of things to do between 3:30 and 5:30 P.M., for example. The individualized plan may be to exercise between 3:30 and 4:00 P.M., to do homework between 4 and 5 P.M., and to watch a favorite TV show between 5:30 and 6 P.M. From 6 to 6:30 P.M. your child can do other chores around the house. The objective is to substitute sitting in front of the TV set and snacking in the afternoon for some other constructive behaviors. Setting up a definite schedule helps.

Lester, for example, found the period between homework time and exercise time on his schedule very difficult. So his mother got him a hard jigsaw puzzle that he loved to work on. Mary, on the other hand, found that 8 P.M., when her brother and sister were having their snacks, was a most difficult time. She suggested, on her own, that she save her fruit salad or call a friend or read that special book she enjoys during the problem time.

Other children find the most difficult time to resist temptation when they watch TV or wait for dinner. Many have found that during those vulnerable times, anything that involves handwork is good—crocheting, model building, handicrafts, or even playing solitaire. Others have found that eating their salads before dinner helps or just taking a big drink of water or broth takes the edge off the hunger.

Weekends are a difficult time and again the idea is to

have a tight schedule planned. If the problem time is Saturday afternoon, your child could arrange going into town with a friend, visiting a hobby shop or toy store or magazine store. Of course, your child should try to avoid the ice cream parlor, candy store, or bakery. If they can buy something that will last and bring it home instead of eating while out that helps reinforce determination to control weight.

Many families, of course, use the weekend to eat out as a recreation. If yours does, try to select restaurants that offer calorie controllable food. However, if possible, it would be good to substitute another family activity for the weekend such as an outing to the ball park or just a walk in a town park. Food celebrations associate pleasant emotions with feasting, a difficult connection to break.

There is usually a lot of open time on Sunday afternoon. A hike with the family or just tossing a Frisbee outside provides emotional food and fun that are not connected to eating. If it is raining, why not pursue a family activity such as a board game like Monopoly or Trivial Pursuit, which take a lot of time, or a card game?

The more time you can spend with your child, the more he will be reassured you love him and are interested in his welfare—and he will be away from food.

CHAPTER V

TEMPTATION TIMES— HOLIDAYS, PARTIES, VACATIONS, OUTINGS

Jack, a popular redhead, was always invited to a lot of parties.

"I used to eat three pieces of cake and as much ice cream and candy as I could get," eleven-year-old Jack recalled. "It was very hard for me when I decided to go to Thin Kids. I thought I would have to give up going to parties. Now I take just one piece of cake and eat it without the icing. I skip the candy because I know if I eat just one, I'll eat a lot. I take half the ice cream and then skip a milk and bread to make up for the party. I also ask to leave the table and go and play with some of the presents that the kid whose party it is got."

We know that birthday and holiday parties offer terrible temptations to children and that is why your youngster needs your help to fortify his defenses. Your child can, if he knows a party is on the schedule for the day, save up a bread and milk, as Jack did. You can also speak to the hosts and inform them that your child is trying to eat different kinds of food. Ask if your youngster can bring a low calorie treat or a bag of fruit to be shared if none will be served.

Your child can eat before she goes to the party. That's a great hint for an adult who also wishes to control food intake. If you are not hungry when you go to a party, you will not be as tempted to dump your food plan.

Discuss with your child before the party what he can do while the other kids are eating cake and ice cream. Can he dance? Play a game? Play with the family pet?

If your child does not want to be away from the table during the festivities, she can eat plain ice cream for the day's milk allowance, if ice cream becomes an important desire. Your child can also eat a piece of cake without the icing but warn her that she will probably feel like eating the icing too, once one bite is taken.

If it is a pizza party, your child can skip the breads for that day and then have one slice of a regular pizza and another with just the cheese. Your child can donate something to the party such as popcorn, a popular but not fattening treat (without the butter, of course).

VALENTINE'S DAY

Just as birthday parties and school parties are difficult times for a child trying to control a weight problem, holidays can sabotage even the strongest of defenses unless you help your child cope.

Jennifer got a big candy heart on Valentine's Day with those small fun messages on them. But for Jennifer the message was "Forget your diet. Candy means love." The heart is a symbol of love, indeed, but there are other ways to show love without calories. A Valentine's card, for example, a chocolate fruit heart or a small present. Flowers, stickers, a charm for a bracelet or necklace, are some valentines that have gone over well with members of our Thin Kids groups.

HALLOWEEN

This is probably the most difficult holiday for a child trying to stick to a food plan. Almost all kids love the fun of begging candy. Instead, you could have a party at your house with healthy snacks such as apples and popcorn and traditional games such as dunking for apples, eating a marshmallow on a string, and pin the tail on the donkey. As part of the holiday fun, you can bake pumpkin seeds on a Teflon cookie tray with a little salt. In this day and age it is safer all around to have at-home parties for children on Halloween. But if your youngster still wants to go begging with friends give him some snacks to take along such as raisins, popcorn, an apple, a fruit drink, sugarless gum, or carrot and celery sticks. The walking around the neighborhood could be a benefit. Think of it as exercise and having a good time with friends. You could buy back the candy with which your child returns with coins and then either throw out the candy or give it to a worthy cause. (That doesn't mean you. Some parents gain a lot of weight eating their children's Halloween candy.) As for what you give out at your own home, raisins, coins, apples, or some small token is better than candy for neighborhood children. If you still want to give out candy, it is wiser not to have your child be the one to hand it out. If any candy is left over, get rid of it before it proves too much of a temptation in the house.

CHRISTMAS—FILL THE STOCKING WITH SENSE AND CENTS

Emphasize the family meaning rather than the feasting as the main part of holiday celebrations. Christmas dinner usually consists of meat, vegetables, salad, and potato, and the menu does not have to be high calorie if the dishes are prepared with more basic recipes. The dessert can be a special fruit salad, low calorie ice cream, or sherbet.

If your child is going to have the meal at a relative's house, talk to the host to find out what kind of food will be served. If it is an understanding relative, the host will make sure that there are foods available your child can eat. If not, bring along or send the right kind of meal for your youngster.

TEMPTATION TIMES

If you know the relative who is a food pusher is going to be present, try to arrange it so that your child does not sit near him or her at the dinner table. (See Chapter VI.) It would also be a good idea for you to sit next to your child at the table so you can give support, encouragement, and guidance quietly during the meal.

Your child's Christmas stocking, of course, should not be filled with candy. You can put little toys, clothing items, and coupon cards that say such things as "Good for One Free Trip to the Zoo" or "Good for One Game of Monopoly" in it. You also can put toys, sugarless gum, baseball cards, stickers, fruits, raisins, or just about anything that is not full of calories in it too.

HANUKKAH—A TREAT FOR EVERY NIGHT

This holiday is not as associated with feasting as many. There are candies and cakes associated with it but the little gifts that children love and the stories that are told are the emphasis. However, it is wise to be vigilant and help your child deal with the temptations put before them by well meaning relatives.

EASTER—DON'T HIDE FROM THE BUNNY

Holiday lamb and ham will not throw off a child's diet too much if the youngster is given a small portion and the food is prepared without the sweet trimmings. The big temptation during this holiday is the Easter basket. Make sure you fill your child's with non-caloric treats. Instead of spending a lot of money on the commercial candy-filled baskets, think of some creative things to put in there. You could get a small jigsaw puzzle, for example, or a Frisbee or new ball—since Easter heralds spring and time outdoors after the winter. You also could include a cheese rabbit, sugarless gum, sugarless candy, raisins, nuts, a colorful bag of popcorn.

PASSOVER—DOES NOT MEAN PASSING UP THE TRADITIONAL FOOD

Emphasize the hunt for the matzo and give a good present because the Seder meal is a challenge. Your child will certainly need your help to keep to the food program while enjoying the traditional meal. A matzo can be exchanged for a bread. Your child can eat one matzo ball instead of a bread and fat. The chicken broth is fine. It is a good idea for your child to skip breads during the whole day. As for the chopped liver—well, that is high in fat but you can prepare it with just enough fat to make it stay together. The gefilte fish is fine with some horseradish. The turkey or brisket, salad and vegetables are all good. A small portion of kugel and stuffing is all right, but again no bread for the day. Fruits for dessert or sherbet is fine.

THANSKGIVING—BE THANKFUL FOR THE FOOD PROGRAM

Turkey is great for your child's program. It is low in calories and it is the main part of the meal. In fact, Thanksgiving is one of the easiest of the holidays because plenty of turkey is available, as well as sometimes ham or roast beef. Your child should exchange a bread and a fat for a half cup of stuffing for the occasion. Skip the cranberries or have a tablespoon of cranberry sauce. Baked yams are delicious, low in calories, and high in nutrition. You can offer low calorie ice cream or baked apples for dessert. (See recipe on page 199.) Again, the main theme of the holiday should be the family get together and thankfulness for all one's blessings.

TEMPTATION TIMES

RESTAURANTS—THE MENU FOR DOING IT RIGHT

So much of American family celebrations are around eating and eating out that it is difficult to separate emotions and eating. We associate happy times with the family with big, festive meals not only during holidays but on family outings.

Some children say "I'm going out to a restaurant, so I'm not going to eat all day." But by the time the child gets to the restaurant, he is so hungry that he grabs all the bread and starts eating it. It takes the food at least fifteen minutes of preparation before it gets to the table. Urge your child to eat the other two meals of the day but to skip some of the bread and milk allowances.

The choice of restaurant is important because some are easier for those on a food program than others. However, your child can make menu selections wisely in almost any restaurant, with a little preparation beforehand.

In an Italian restaurant, for example, your child could make a delicious meal out of the antipasto and use a slice of pizza as a side dish. Italian salad, or any salad for that matter, is filling. However, if your child's nemesis is lasagna or eggplant parmesan, it would be best to skip the Italian restaurant because it would be harder for her to resist the temptation. But if your child is not enamoured by the above, she can go to an Italian restaurant and very wisely order a veal or chicken dish. If you ask for a child's portion, it will not only be cheaper in money but also it will be cheaper in calories.

CHINESE RESTAURANT—HOLD THE M.S.G.

Start with the egg drop soup but eat just half a bowl. The won ton soup is fine without the won ton. Your child should eat just the inside of the eggroll instead of the outside. He should order white rice instead of fried rice. The roast pork appetizer is better than the spareribs and chicken chow mein or any vegetable dish with chicken or meat is fine. Ask the restaurant to leave out the M.S.G. and cut down on the cornstarch, which adds a lot of unnecessary calories, as much as possible. The restaurant usually offers fruit for dessert, a wise selection, of course.

FRENCH RESTAURANTS—WITHOUT THE SAUCES

The French are good cooks but they do love rich sauces. However, more and more French restaurants are offering lighter meals. Chicken, veal, or fish without the sauce is fine. Ask the chef to cut down on the butter. Your child should probably skip the bread and fat for the day so she can enjoy a piece of French bread and allow for some French touches to the dishes served. Fruit or sherbet for dessert is recommended.

AMERICAN—STARS AND STRIPES

There is great menu freedom in a true blue American restaurant. Your child can select from a wide variety of foods—hamburgers, steaks, chicken—but it is a good idea to discuss the choices with him before looking at the menu because seeing all the dishes listed can be very tempting. Your child can save the bread for the day and eat a hamburger on half a bun or eat it on a plate with lettuce, tomato, and salad, a hot vegetable, and a baked potato. French fries are a no-no and so are other foods that have a lot of mayonnaise and sauces. Your child can let the waiter or waitress know that he is on a special menu plan and ask for suggestions. Most American restaurants have fish, chicken, and steak and the waiter or waitress can request that the chef leave off extra butter. If bread is brought to the table, either request it be taken away or move it away from the child. Your youngster can bring his own low calorie dressing or just ask for oil and vinegar. It is also a good idea to bring a doodle mat or some game to play at the table, because it is usually a *long-g-g* time before the food is served. As for dessert, most American restaurants offer fruits or fruit salad. Sherbet is all right too.

FAST FOOD RESTAURANTS—CAN SERVE A FOOD PROGRAM

Fast food restaurants have a reputation for serving fatty, highly salted foods but that does not have to be the situation for your child. Choose a fast food restaurant that has a lot of variety including *broiled* hamburgers, a salad bar, and other choices such as *broiled chicken* or *fish*. The foods to avoid are potato salad, cole slaw, and high calorie dressings, as well as French fries and other fried foods and those special sauces. Your child can enjoy lots of fresh vegetables: broccoli, cauliflower, carrots, peppers, cucumbers, lettuce, tomatoes, and mushrooms. Many fast food places now serve breakfast, so milk or juice is usually available all day as a beverage. If not, water should be ordered in place of soda. A good meal at a fast food restaurant would be: broiled burger (large size) on half the bun with lettuce, tomato, and pickles and dressed with one tablespoon of catsup mixed with a little mustard. Also salad on the side and a beverage such as juice, milk, or water should accompany the meal. Bring along a fruit for dessert.

ON VACATIONS—TAKE ALONG THE PROGRAM

Children who go to a hotel on a vacation may find it difficult, again, to follow a food plan. You can prepare your child before by discussing wise choices. Once they see the menu and are not prepared, they will most likely be tempted. Fish, chicken, fruits, and vegetables are usually on all menus. If you take this book along and speak to the chef, most will work with you to prepare the right meals for your child.

AT CAMP—STAYING IN THE SWIM OF THINGS

Even if you don't send cookies and other treats to camp, other parents do. Some bunks have a candy trunk in the middle where donations are put in and candy and cookies are taken out at will. Diet- and nutrition-minded camps may help to make your child's summer away a good time for weight loss. The meals often offer second and third helpings, but you can ask your child's counselor to encourage your child to skip seconds. The kitchen aides may also be helpful if you discuss your child's program with them. Snack times may include high calorie foods like cookies, candy, and ice cream, so help out by sending the right care package for your child with enough for other members of the bunk. Include popcorn and some pretzels, low calorie gum, games, puzzles, magazines, and fruit juice. There are also specific diet camps; they do need good follow-up to ensure maintenance. The Thin Kids book can help combat the roller coaster effect of coming back home to the environment that contributed to the excess weight problem in the first place.

MOVIES—THE SHOW MUST GO ON

Make sure your child brings her own treat to the movies. It can be popcorn, fruit, fruit juice, a Thermos bottle of water, raisins, or sugarless gum. Plan in the morning for movies so that the bread and/or fruit can be saved for the occasion. Emphasize the main reason for going to a movie is to see the show. Most people finish their candy before the movie even starts so before the show goes on, encourage your child to go to the lounge or to carry on a conversation before the movie begins. It is a good idea not to have the child sit between two kids or adults who are eating a lot of candy and even passing it back and forth.

In this chapter we have described the occasions that are particularly hard for a child to stick to a food program. But it can be done with a little preplanning, some creativity, and a lot of your support and encouragement.

CHAPTER VI

LOVE WITH CALORIES—DEALING WITH FOOD PUSHERS

There is great emphasis in Western culture in being thin, yet our society does everything to push food on children. Main street is filled with ice cream parlors, fast food restaurants, and candy stores. The commercials, particularly on TV, keep repeating the good taste of highly sugared cereals, fatty fast foods, oily snacks, and candy bars. Holidays with feasts and sweet treats are a part of tradition and widely promoted in the media. But there also are beloved food pushers, particularly among older relatives, who equate giving food with giving love.

As a concerned parent, you can defend your child against the pushers and give him gentle but strong weapons with which to fend off temptation. Your child must learn to stand up for her own rights and say no!

Ralph's grandmother, for example, would cook lavish meals of potatoes, pasta, cakes, and ice cream whenever he stayed with her over the weekend. He loved his grandma and did not want to hurt her feelings by refusing.

Cicely's parents were divorced. She had to cook her own meals because her mother worked until seven P.M. in a store. A latchkey child in the city, she was lonesome and would use food to comfort herself. Her father, to make matters worse, would take Cicely out on the weekends and offer her sundaes, candy, and other sweets he knew she liked.

Cicely's situation is very common in our society. Often divorced parents or even working parents feel guilty and try to make up for their imagined slights to their children with sweet or fattening foods. We, at Thin Kids, understand why they do it but make every effort to point out why they should not. If they really want to show love to an obese child, they should help the youngster deal with the habits and emotions that caused either overeating or improper eating in the first place. Admittedly, it takes more time to go for a walk or play a game with your child than it does to hand her an ice cream cone or a bag of candy, but you will find that the sweets will not last long but the memory of the shared activity will.

We always ask kids in the Thin Kids program who are the food pushers in their lives.

> Number one is usually Grandma or some other relative.
> Number two is friends.
> Number three is Mother or Father.
> Number four is the teacher.

We also ask them to come up with some reasons that people push food. Among the common ones they suggest:

> "People don't like to eat alone."
> "Lots of time your friends and relatives push food on you because they don't think you are eating enough."
> "They think they know better than your doctor knows."
> "They don't want food to go to waste."

We all remember that last one. Didn't your parents tell you "Children are starving in India [or Africa or China]?" Why didn't you tell them that if you ate your spinach, it wouldn't help the starving children?

Ask your child who the food pushers are in her life and discuss why and what will happen if your youngster refuses a preferred treat. For example, if Ralph kept eating with his grandma who didn't like to eat alone, he would keep putting on weight and might be very lonely himself. We try to help children handle the food pushers in their own lives.

Through role playing you—taking the part of the food pusher—and your child can rehearse turning off the insistent tempter. The next time Ralph's grandmother offered him a piece of cake she had just made, he said, "Please, Grandma. Don't offer me cake because you know I'm on a food plan and am trying to lose weight. If you really want to make me happy, help me. Offer me foods that are good for me."

Most grandmas, as Ralph's did, can understand how hard it is for the child and will cooperate if the youngster asks for help.

In Cicely's case it was her divorced father who was the food pusher. She, too, pointed out to him the true situation.

"Dad," she told him, "the kids at school have been giving me a hard time and a lot of them call me names. So I need you to help me lose weight so that the kids will stop."

She asked her father to take her for a hike instead of to the ice cream store, as he did each week. She also asked him to take her to another place to eat.

"Can't we go to a restaurant that will be easier for me to get the foods that won't make me fatter?" Cicely asked him.

Her dad told us that he really did not realize that instead of helping his daughter and showing his love, he was doing something that was making her unhappy all week long. He came to class one evening with her because she really got to him when she said, "You don't see me during the week when I come home crying after school."

Both Ralph's grandmother and Cicely's father did help their children once they fully understood that there are other ways to show love rather than through giving a youngster fattening food. The youngsters, on the other hand, learned how to say no to an adult they loved without hurting the adult's feelings.

Saying no to one's peers, however, may be even more difficult. Shari liked Cindy and wanted to be her friend so she found it very difficult to say no when Cindy invited her to come with the other kids and eat cookies in the cafeteria.

Shari could understand that Cindy kept insisting that they

go and eat cookies together because she wanted to share the activity with her friend. Instead, Shari could ask Cindy to go in the yard and jump rope or go to the classroom and paint pictures. That still would involve two friends sharing an activity together.

On the other hand Shari's friend Betty had a different reason for urging Shari to eat cookies. She knew Shari was on a diet and, because of some "hurt" in her own life, she wanted to see Shari "breakdown" and eat the cookies. Children can understand other children feeling jealous or competitive and trying to undermine a food program. Talking about it helps armor your child against such attacks.

Many times, however, friends just want to share good times with a child and they and/or their parents are not aware that they are sabotaging a diet. If your child is invited to a friend's house for dinner, your child or you could explain to the youngster's family that your child is on a food program. Most parents are very willing to cooperate. If it is too much trouble or the food is already prepared and is unsuitable, your youngster could then take his or her own meal to eat with the friend.

In the Thin Kids program we do skits in which a child plays the part of either the food pusher or the one being tempted.

This is really a rehearsal for reality. You can do these informal skits with your youngster. Together you can portray the reasons food is pushed and the best way to refuse in various circumstances. Here are some common situations a child may face.

The Sleep Over

A lot of snacks will be offered. Ask your child how he or she will refuse the cookies and pretzels and potato chips offered. Could he say, "I'm thirsty. May I have a glass of water?" "Can I look over your records [or games]?" Your child, of course, could bring his own snacks. In all these skits encourage your youngster to think up her own solutions.

Eating at a Relative's House

A grandmother or aunt may cook up your child's favorite dishes of the past such as ravioli or fudge. Sometimes

LOVE WITH CALORIES

they will be very insistent or very disappointed if your child refuses the food. Grandma may have baked an apple pie and might say, "Eat it, it's good for you. It has apples in it." Your child might say, "But what about the sugar?" Grandma may respond, "Oh, a little bit won't hurt." Or she may show great disappointment that your child won't accept the treat. Therefore, it is much better to call in advance and ask a relative that a steak and salad or chicken be prepared instead, and fruit be offered for dessert instead of pie, ice cream, and/or cookies. If that is impractical, then your child can learn to eat just a little portion. Saying "Thank you, but I'm not hungry" will often help turn off the food pusher, and if that doesn't work, "Thank you, but my doctor told me not to eat it." That is true if the pediatrician or family doctor has recommended a weight loss. Many people would not urge a diabetic child to eat sweets, yet they do not hesitate to urge an overweight child to eat something fattening.

Calories in Sibling Rivalry

It is common for a sibling to utilize a brother or sister's weight problem as a means of maintaining superiority. You have to help your child combat your other child or children's efforts to sabotage by teasing and tempting. We think you will be quite surprised by the hidden feelings that emerge when you and your child play out the sibling rivalry in your home.

The School Party

You and your child can take the parts of the school food pusher—it may be the homeroom mother or a friend or the teacher—and the part of the resister. It will be fun to make up the skit together and it will prepare your child to meet the challenges in the real world. For example, a friend may offer a cupcake. Your child might say, "No, thanks. I had a big lunch [or breakfast]." The friend may say, "Oh, a few crumbs won't hurt you." Ask your child what he would answer. Again, the idea is to get your child to think up his own solutions.

Youngsters soon learn to develop their own techniques. For example, Nancy, a thirteen-year-old, tells people who offer her candy or cake, "No, thanks, I'm allergic."

"If I say I'm on a diet, they just keep urging me to take a little piece or they say 'One piece won't hurt you,' " Nancy explained.

Jean, eight, whose mother at first had to urge her to attend sessions of Thin Kids, developed her own special method to turn off food pushers.

"I just imagine that I am offered *poison!* And then I am not tempted."

That must work because Jean lost sixteen pounds.

Mary, a pretty thirteen-year-old blonde who came to Thin Kids on her own, said, "I have learned to tune myself into something else whenever I'm tempted. For example, this summer we joined a swim club. I just knew I'd be tempted by its fast food place if I sat around all day. So I got myself a job as a baby-sitter to keep busy. And when I feel like binging, like I used to do, I just run it off."

It becomes easier to resist temptation. Mary, the daughter of a railroad engineer, explained, "I had always been last in the races at school. We recently had a quarter mile race and I came in third. I heard one of the kids say, 'Hey, what's Mary doing coming in third. She's always last!' I felt great inside."

John, a green-eyed, curly haired twelve-year-old who wanted to lose weight because he wants to be a professional baseball player, had his own techniques. A very handsome fellow, the girls at school were all in love with him. He lost twelve pounds and became the star hitter of his Little League baseball team.

"The girls at school offer me corn chips and other fattening stuff but I tell myself, John, you'll only be cheating yourself. So I say, 'No, thanks!' I used to eat four slices of cake at a birthday party. Now I just eat a salad or do something besides eating, like playing a game. We celebrate everytime my dad has to punch another hole in my belt because it's too big."

The family of twelve-year-old Lucy likes to go to the ball park where they eat hotdogs (salty and fatty) and drink soda (full of sugar).

"We still go to the ball park," Lucy laughed, "but I bring my own treats—usually fruit."

Once it is clear to your child that you know how difficult

it is to refuse, especially if more than one friend is pushing, and that rehearsing together various situations will be of great help, chances are that the defenses built by the two of you will hold strong.

A Child's Imagination Can Be a Wonderous Thing

Another technique, that is sort of a rehearsal in mind only, is the use of imagery. You can help your child to use mind pictures or happy predictions of the future to resist food pushers and other temptations. For example, tell your child to close her eyes and imagine that she has lost a lot of weight and is meeting a relative or friend for the first time with a new shape. Ask your youngster to think of all the good things that may occur. Being better at sports, looking better, feeling better, buying the clothes she wants.

Sticking to a sensible food program is hard work as we all know. But with rehearsal and imagination, your child has techniques that will help ease the way. They will help prepare your child not only for childhood food temptations but for adult ones, later on.

CHAPTER VII

FIGHTING FAT WITH FUN AND GAMES

One of the greatest gifts you can give your kids is making exercise an ingrained habit. As a parent, you know that proper exercise is an excellent and quick way to improve health and appearance. People who are physically active have half the heart disease rate of people who are not. Folks who just "sit around" have a greater incidence of diabetes, ulcers, and other internal ailments. Furthermore, an estimated eighty percent of the cases of low back pain can be traced to lack of physical exercise. Repeated experiments have shown that exercise improves the action of the heart, blood circulation, and breath. It improves muscle tone and certainly helps control weight. It not only burns up calories, it dampens appetite and the boredom that often leads to eating.

In the late 1950s and 1960s, the President's Council on Physical Fitness found that many children were not physically fit. Since then physical education has taken on a new direction and has become more sensitive to the needs of the individual and attempts are made to provide a child with remedial training. Nevertheless, the amount of exercise a child gets in school is minimal, especially after the cutbacks in school budgets in recent years. Therefore you, as a parent, will have to use your ingenuity to get your youngster up and moving.

Sometimes it is simple. Drew, for example, wanted to make the soccer team in the worst way. He was overweight, so we advised him to start walking and kicking a ball against a wall for at least half an hour per day. In a month's time he lost a little weight and his coordination and endurance improved dramatically. He made the team and after a few months of going to scheduled practices and competition, he was down to normal weight.

On the other hand, we have seen overweight children (not at Thin Kids, of course) who want to make a team go on crash diets and even sit on radiators to lose weight. So they do need adult guidance.

Certainly, not all overweight children are all poor athletes. Some are excellent and even welcome the weight in order to play certain sports, such as football. As long as these heavyweights are active, they have no problem. But, after high school or college when they are no longer part of a football team, they can become very overweight.

A broken arm or sickness can sometimes immobilize a child and produce a weight problem. But for the most part, as we have pointed out throughout the book, a weight problem is mostly due to too much food and too little activity. What if your child is not motivated and/or does not know of any exercise that is appealing. How can you help?

First of all, discuss with your child the benefits of exercise. A dramatic and effective technique is to hand your youngster a bag of groceries of approximately the same poundage that your child is overweight. Ask your child to carry the bundle up and down the stairs twice and then explain that is an example of how much strain overweight puts on his body. And point out how much faster he will be able to do everything without that extra bruden.

Then, together, you can discuss the various possibilities of sports and physical activities that your child might like. Your attitude, effort, and guidance are vital to help your youngster derive the maximum physical and psychological benefits of any activity.

One of the great incentives many children have for losing weight is that they do want to become more athletic so they can participate in more sports. If your child feels that way, you are already ahead of the game. But what sport would offer the best physical benefits?

Physical fitness consists of three basic components.

1. **Strength.** This is what kids consider fitness. But what is strength for one child, may be weakness for another. It is very important, of course, for your youngster to develop and maintain muscles.
2. **Endurance.** Your child can be strong but have no endurance. A youngster should be able to maintain physical activity for a reasonable period of time to be considered fit.
3. **Flexibility.** A child should have good tone and litheness in his or her muscles, particularly of the lower back and abdomen.

Here are some simple—but not infallible tests—for your child to determine just how fit she is.

FITNESS TEST

- Stand on one foot, like a stork. Close your eyes and with your hands on hips, try to hold this position while counting to fifteen. (If your child can do this without falling over, he is in at least fair physical condition.)
- Lie on the floor on your stomach, arms stretched out in front and head down. Raise your right arm and left leg, then your left arm and right leg. The legs and arms should not touch the floor for at least one minute. If your child can do this without straining, his endurance is pretty good.
- Bend over while the feet are two inches apart and touch the ankles without bending the knees.
- Crawl thirty feet on your stomach using only the elbows as a means of propulsion and no leg movement whatsoever. The child over twelve years should be able to crawl at least forty feet.
- Jump rope. From age eight to ten, thirty to fifty times with feet together without missing a turn. From eleven

to fourteen, seventy-five to one hundred, and from fifteen to eighteen, 150 times.

If your child can perform all of the above, he is reasonably fit and can pursue more vigorous training. However, it is certainly sensible to pursue any exercise program slowly and to build up to it. If there is pain, shortness of breath, or any significant physical symptom, the exercise program should be stopped until a physician is consulted.

Some children do need more exercise than others. The mesomorphs (those with a large muscle mass and large bones) need more physical activity to be in shape and maintain normal weight. The ectomorphs (those with slender skeletons and long, narrow hands and feet) can sit down all day and not get fat. Their appetite is lower, and if they become less mobile, their appetite continues to drop.

Children need aerobic exercise—exercise that raises the pulse rate to seventy to eighty percent of capacity and increases oxygen to the blood. Running in place about eighty beats to a minute, for example, provides aerobic exercise for a child. To gain stamina, a child has to train for endurance. That means she has to huff and puff.

There are children who do not like to sweat. You can tell yours that sweat indicates whether your heart and lungs are going into that aerobic state and burning up calories as well as puts a healthy stress on the heart and lungs. Each time they do that, they will be stronger and be able to do it longer. It is not unusual, however, for body temperature to rise as high as 102 degrees after exercise. Be careful that your child is not overdressed during exercise. It is best to have a child wear layers of clothing that can be peeled off as the body heats up. A word of caution: it is dangerous for a kid who is not in top physical condition—particularly an obese youngster—to exercise in hot humid weather. In any weather, of course, plenty of fluids should be available to replenish water lost through sweating. Plain water is fine. No salt and no fancy drinks for athletes are necessary or wise.

There is enjoyment to working hard and feeling good. There is a sense of fun and accomplishment. Aerobic endurance means that you burn more oxygen, fats, and sugars from your muscle and your liver.

Your child might like to learn how to take his pulse by placing a finger over the carotid artery along either side of the throat. With the thumb on the side of the chin, the fingers will reach the point of the carotid artery along the opposite side of the throat. The pulse can also be taken at a point on the underside of the wrist just below the base of the thumb or by simply placing the hand over the heart. After a workout, if your child counts the number of beats for six seconds and then multiplies by ten, that is his pulse rate for a minute. The objective of training for physical fitness is to achieve seventy to eighty-five percent of the maximal heart rate. To figure that out, subtract your child's age from 220. For example, suppose your child is sixteen years old. Then seventy-five percent of 204 would be about 153 beats per minute. That is the target for vigorous exercise training, but, of course, only if your child has no serious health problems and has regular physical checkups by a physician.

Speed is another thing kids can understand. If they run fast and learn to react quickly, it will help them at sports. Tennis and basketball, for example, help children build up reactions. Agility, coordination, and balance are helped by sports such as gymnastics.

Archery, on the other hand, is not aerobic and has little physical exercise potential. But if a child likes it, it is good for hand-eye coordination and the strength of the arm and chest muscles.

Lou's favorite sport in high school and college was fencing. He was state champion and a national competitor. Fencing is a good physical fitness sport involving aerobic exercise, agility, reaction time, and fun. Children as young as seven or eight can learn fencing. Face masks and protective jackets are essential and so is proper instruction.

Your primary goal should be to expose your child to as many sports as possible. Children under nine years of age have a relatively short attention span so they need variety to stay alert and motivated; sampling a range of activities initially can help them decide on a specialty later on.

But a word of caution: just because your child wants to play a particular sport does not mean he or she is equipped emotionally or physically to do it. It has been reported that volleyball is a risk for children under nine, for example, because bone structure is not totally developed and the stress on the bones and joints can be damaging. You can suggest, instead, playing with a nerf or beach ball or other creative games with a ball. Gymnastics is another activity that should be approached with caution. Although children do start young today, injury can result, especially from the long horse where the full weight of the body comes down.

If your child is awkward, lack of coordination should not be an excuse for not participating in sports. Physical activity is the best way to help your youngster overcome such problems. However, you and your child's teachers have to be sensitive to the difficulties that may occur and see that your youngster is not subjected to ridicule. For example, the biggest crime that can be committed in physical education—and unfortunately it is all too common—is to appoint two captains and have them pick individuals for their teams. Mindy still can feel the hurt of always being the last one chosen, and if your child is overweight, she probably has had the same experience. The YMCA's and YWCA's are very conscious of this and in most such programs, everyone plays. Teams are either pre-determined or randomly selected. If your child's teacher does not do the same, you should try and raise the educator's consciousness.

What are the best exercise choices? Any activity can help a child lose weight. Running, of course, is one of the fastest ways, but any very active sport like swimming or touch football can also be beneficial. The best age for tennis is between eight and eleven years. Tennis is a complicated skill and if your child shows a great deal of interest in it, there will be time to strive for a realistic goal. Starting even younger is all right if your child is eager to do so, but it really doesn't give any extra advantage.

As we pointed out at the beginning of this chapter, your attitude is very important, even if you don't express it in words. If you place too much emphasis on winning, your child may find it difficult to distinguish between being an inadequate player and being an inadequate person. Self-esteem may suffer and your kid might be driven to cheating to protect himself or herself from the disgrace of losing and the fear of incurring your disapproval. It can be frightening for a child to think that a win or loss will affect your love. You have to

assure your child that you love him no matter how he plays.
Try to find a sport that your child will be able to participate in and will be eager to do so. Here are some of the advantages of common sports.

Jogging

The biggest advantage of jogging for kids is the development of proper body alignment and coordination of arm and leg movements. Starting young—with the proper heel-to-toe gait—can prevent foot, leg, hip, and lower back problems. Your child should wear waffle-soled shoes, which provide support and prevent slipping. If your child takes to this sport, he will have toned hamstrings, flexibility, endurance, cardiovascular fitness, and rhythm. Before beginning any workout, of course, a warm-up period consisting of mild stretching, walking, or slow jogging is highly recommended. Warm-ups help to prevent soreness and injury. It also prevents the circulatory system from being shocked by sudden exertions. A cool down at the end of the workout is also very important. Suddenly stopping vigorous exercise may affect the circulatory system and cause the child to become dizzy or even faint.

When starting a jogging program, there should be forty seconds of jogging (about one hundred yards), walking for one minute (about one hundred yards), and repeated nine times for a week. The second week your child can jog for one minute (150 yards), walk one minute (one hundred yards), and repeat that eight times. The third week she can jog two minutes (three hundred yards), walk one minute (one hundred yards), and repeat that six times. The fourth week jog four minutes (six hundred yards), walk one minute (one hundred yards), and repeat four times. The fifth week jog six minutes (nine hundred yards), walk one minute (one hundred yards), and repeat three times. By the sixth week your child should be able to jog eight minutes (1,200 yards), walk two minutes (two hundred yards), and repeat that two times. By the seventh week your youngster should be able to jog ten minutes (1,500 yards), walk two minutes (two hundred yards), repeated two times. And by the eighth week jog twelve minutes (1,700 yards), walk two minutes (two hundred yards), and repeat that two times. Of course, if your child has any pain in the ankles, shins, or chest, she should not jog again until checked by a physician. Be sure that you supervise the place where your child runs. A track at school or in the park is certainly preferable to hard sidewalks or dangerous streets.

Gymnastics

This requires a lot of strength, endurance, and balance. Girls have a special advantage because they are naturally loose-limbed and flexible. Between the ages of ten and fifteen, their bodies are in peak condition for sophisticated power-packed moves. Developing strength, agility, and rhythm may be hard at first for a very overweight child. Make sure the instructor who teaches your child gymnastics is qualified to do so and that the equipment is kept in good order. Gymnastics, unlike tennis or golf, is seldom a life-time sport but can be a great way to teach a child grace and conditioning.

EXERCISE TASKS FOR THIN KIDS

The following program is a challenge and fun for most children and adults. Make a copy of the exercise diary in the next chapter and try to have your child do as many of the following as possible each day, *gradually* building up until she can do all the repetitions within the time specified. You may want to discuss a reward that the child may obtain when she can do all the exercises easily. The biggest reward, of course, will be a sleeker shape. The whole family may also join in and reap the benefits.

THIN KIDS

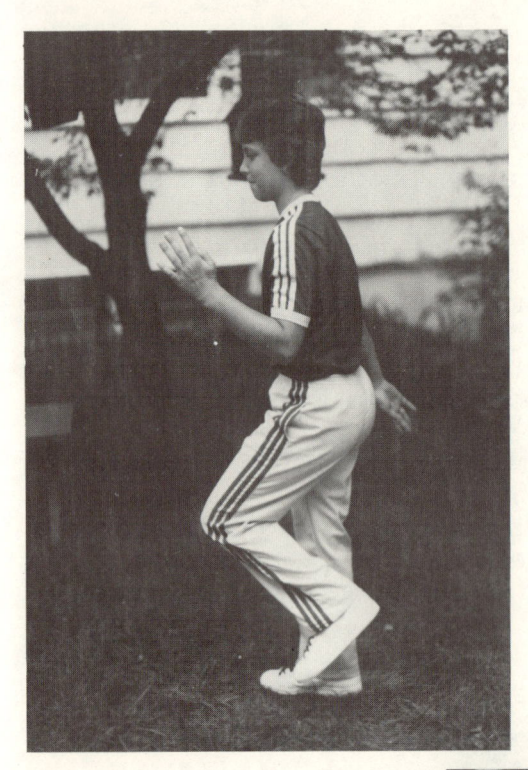

Walk 10 minutes.

Run in place for 3 minutes. This is a good general warm-up.

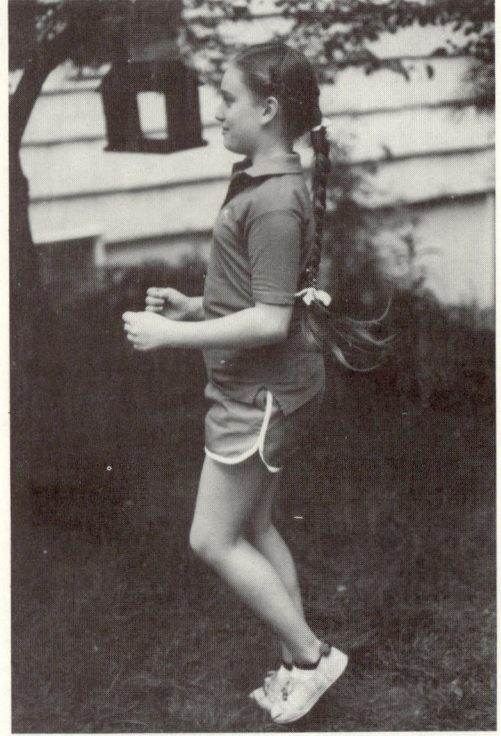

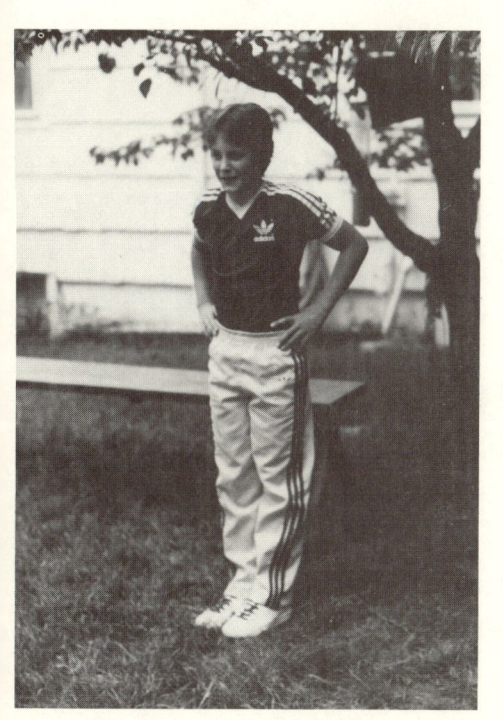

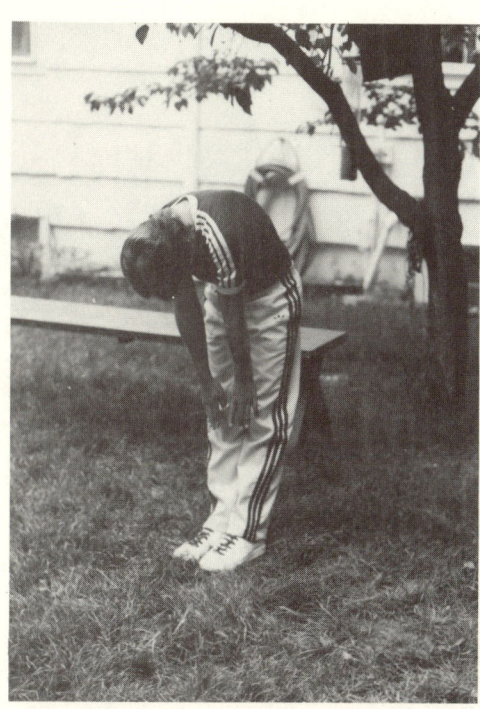

Touch toes 10 times and then reach up 10 times.

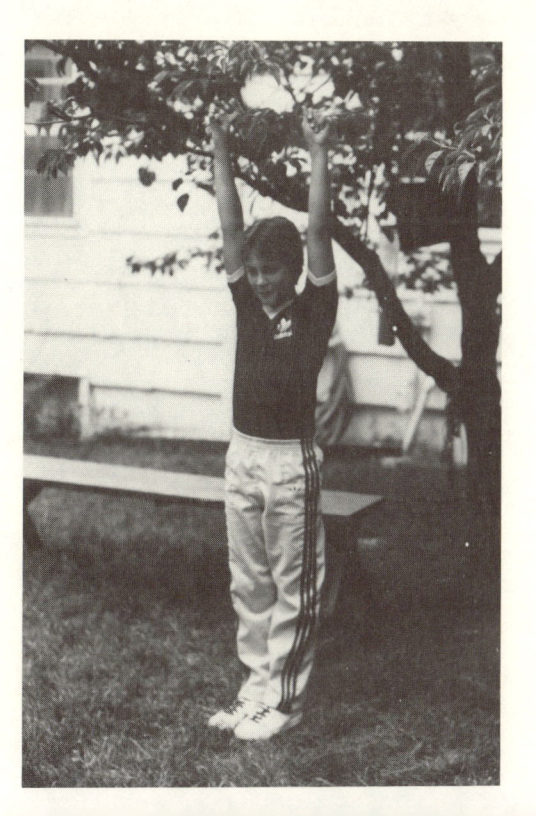

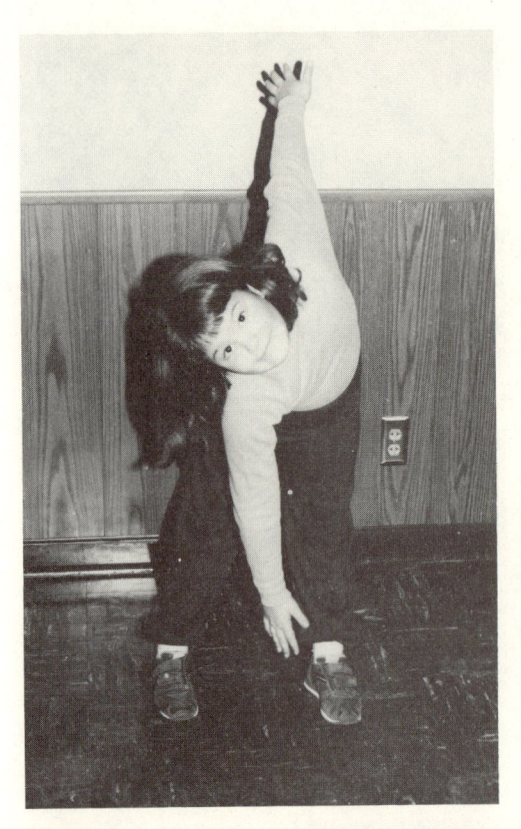

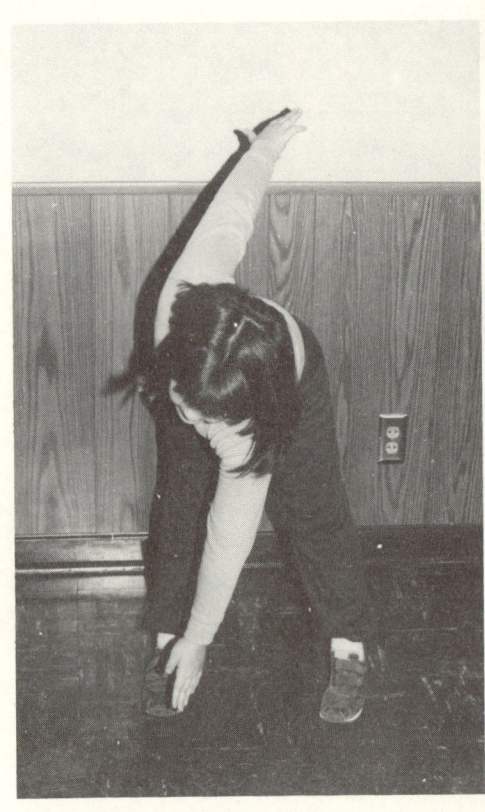

Windmill toe touch 20 times.

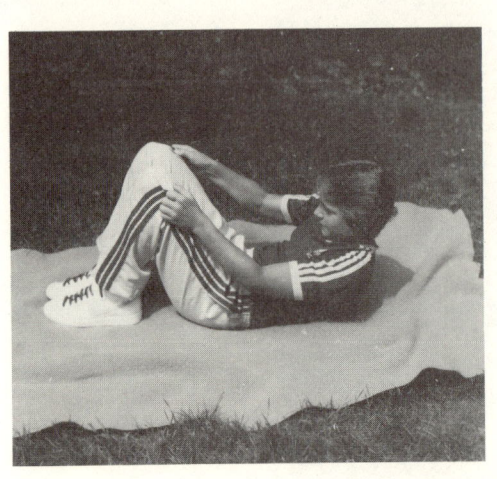

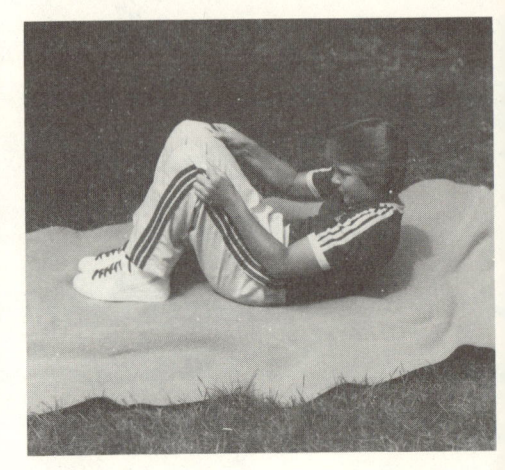

Contract stomach muscles 5 times.

FIGHTING FAT

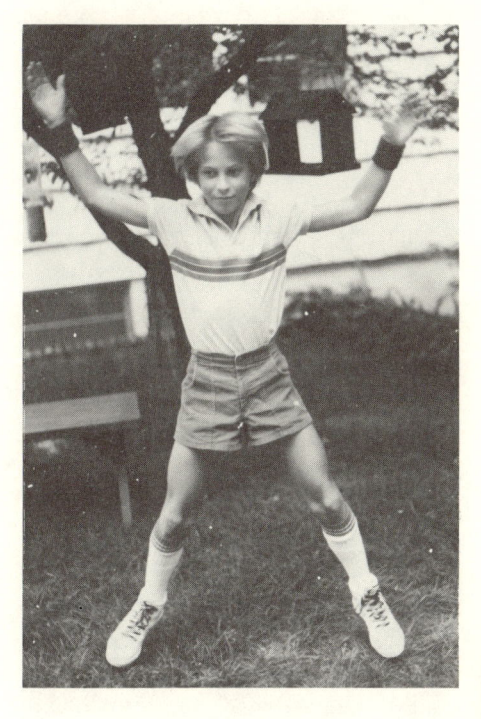

Do jumping jacks for 5 minutes.

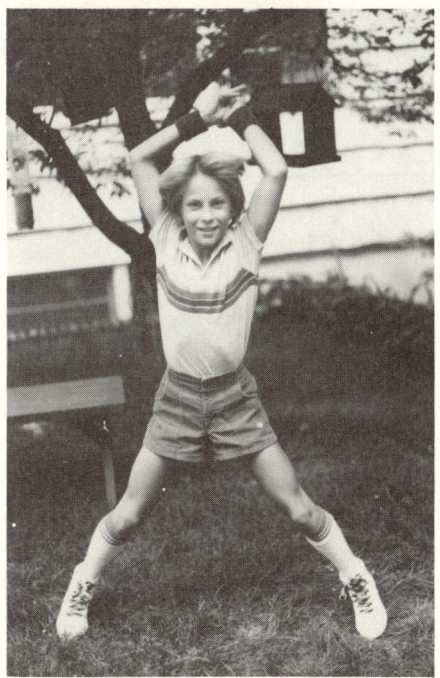

THIN KIDS

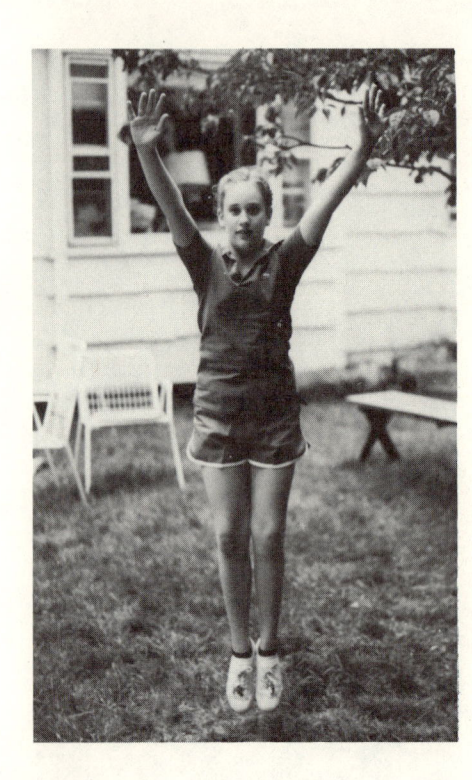

With feet together, jump 5 times.

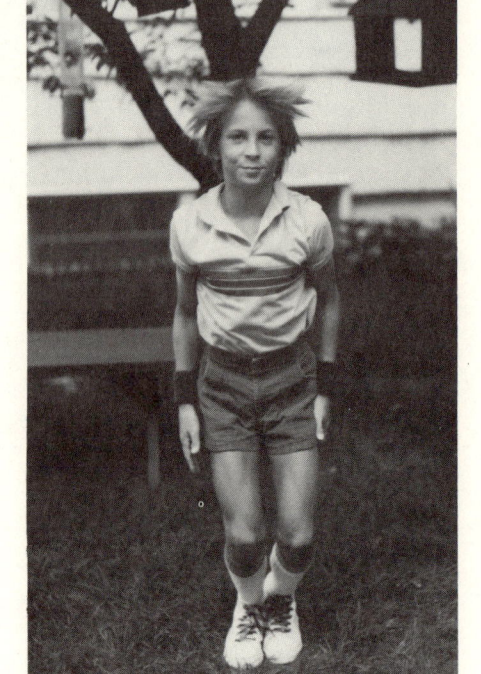

Jump to the sides, snapping legs together in air 10 times.

FIGHTING FAT

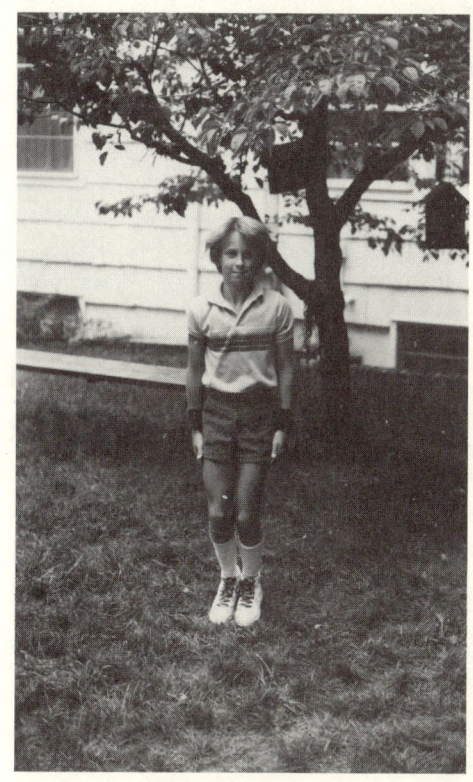

Bounce up and down for 1 minute.

With arms held straight out to the side, do 5 small arm circles, then 5 medium, and 5 large, then, reverse directions and do 5 small, 5 medium, and 5 large.

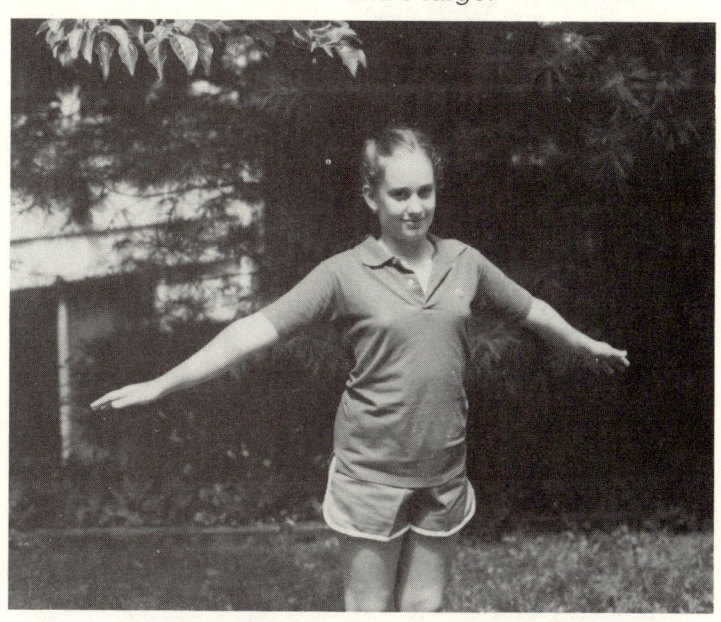

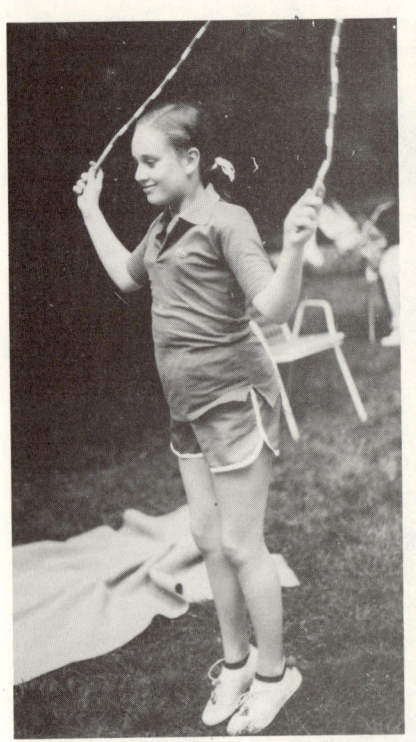

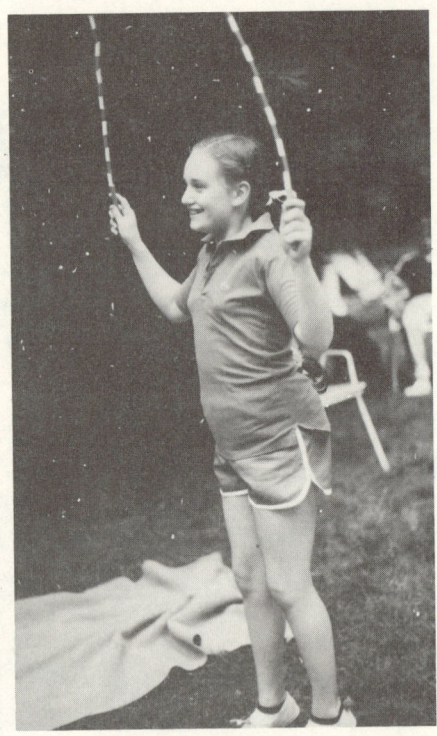

Jump rope 30 seconds and rest. Do this 3 times.

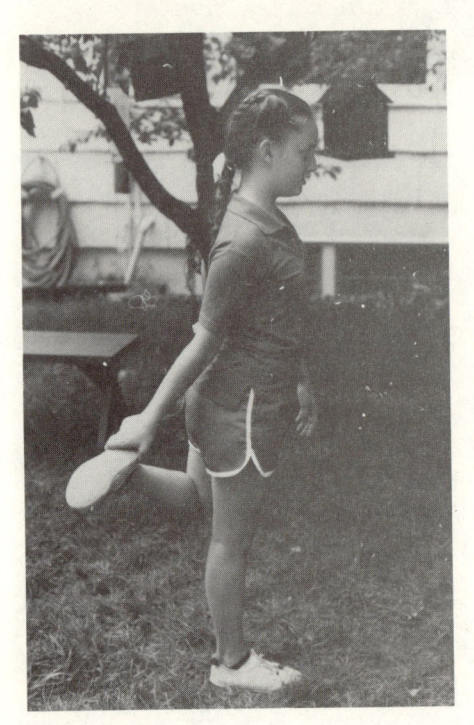

Bend backward and touch right heel with left hand and vice versa.

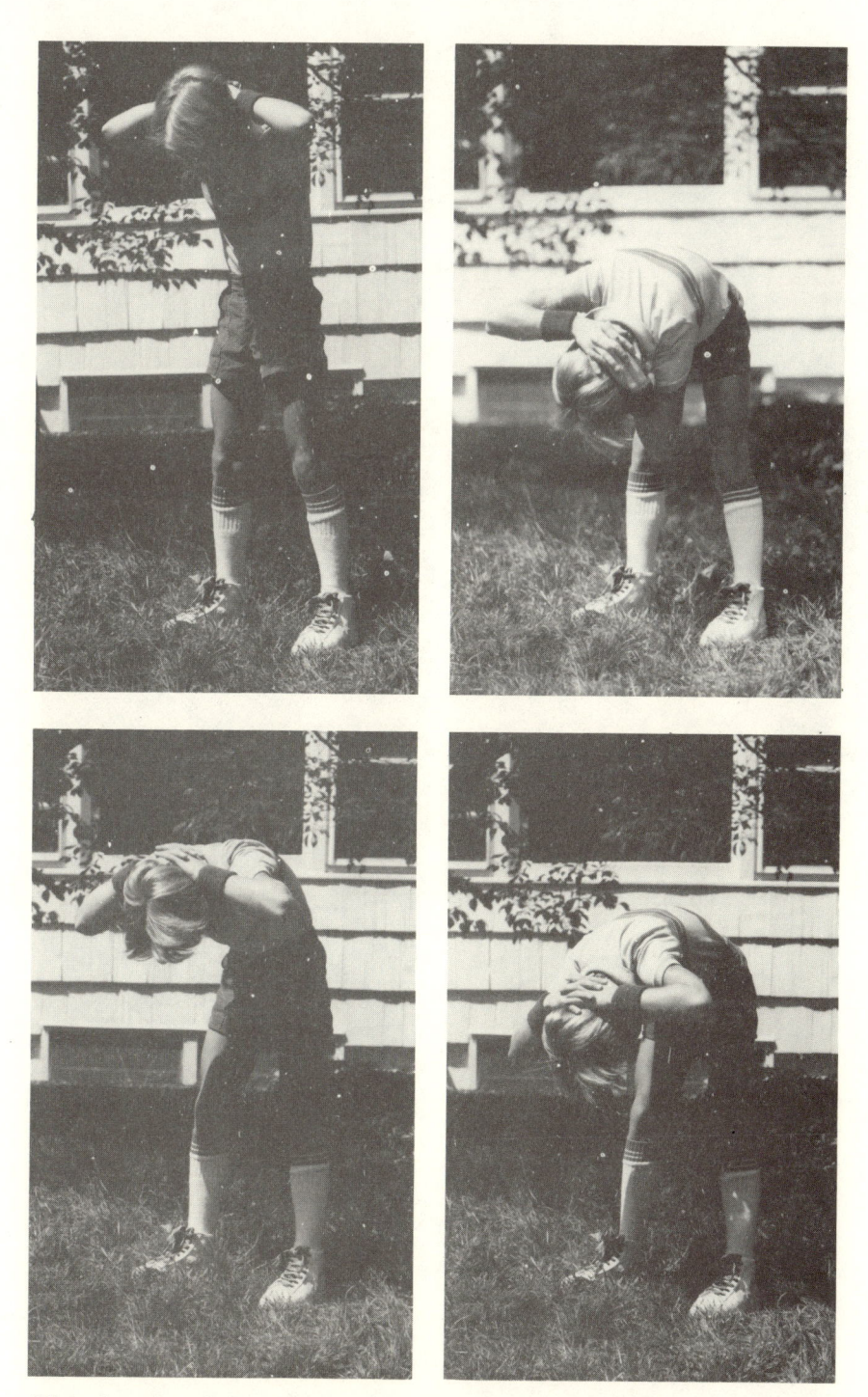

With hands clasped behind head and feet separated about a shoulder width apart, bend forward to waist level and twist trunk to left and then to right and return to starting position.

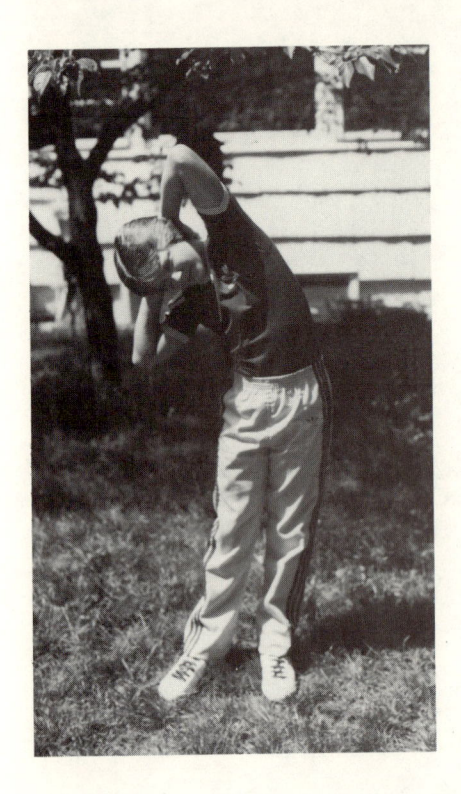

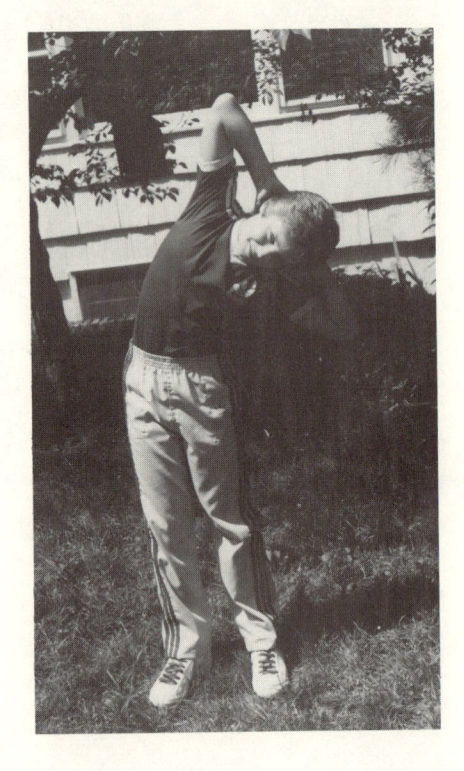

Stand with feet about a shoulder width apart and interlace hands behind head with the elbows back. Bend trunk sideways to the left as far as possible and return to starting position and then bend trunk to right as far as possible and return.

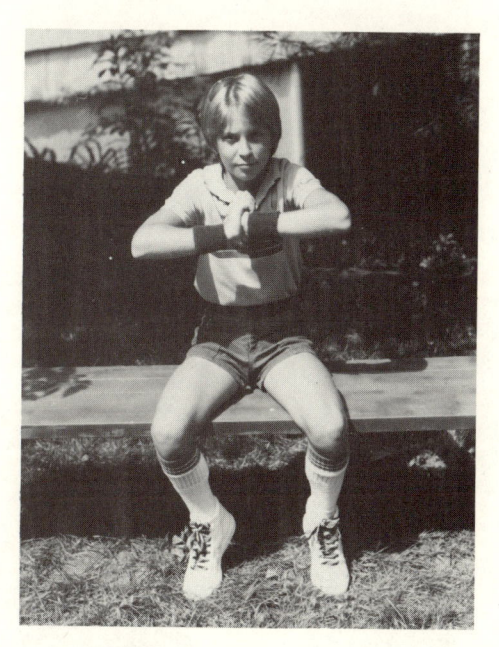

Bend arms across the chest. Place one hand inside the other and press the hands together as hard as possible and hold for 5 seconds. Repeat five times.

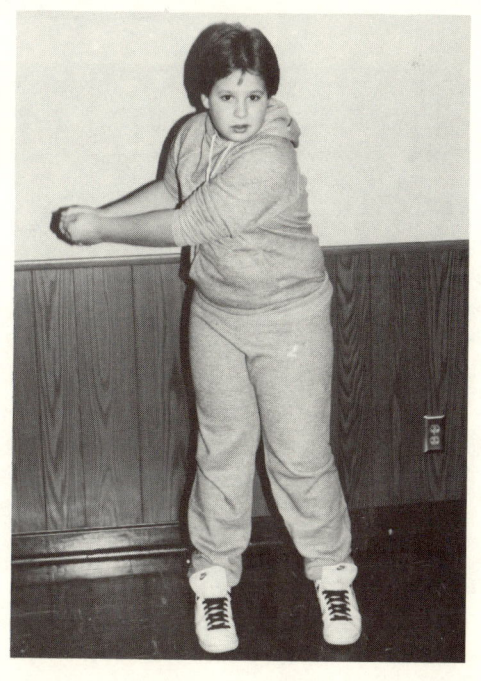

Practice large golf swings for 20 strokes.

Sit in chair, arms at side. Place your hands under your knees and breathe out while pulling up as hard as possible with arms and hands, as if to lift the body up by the chair.

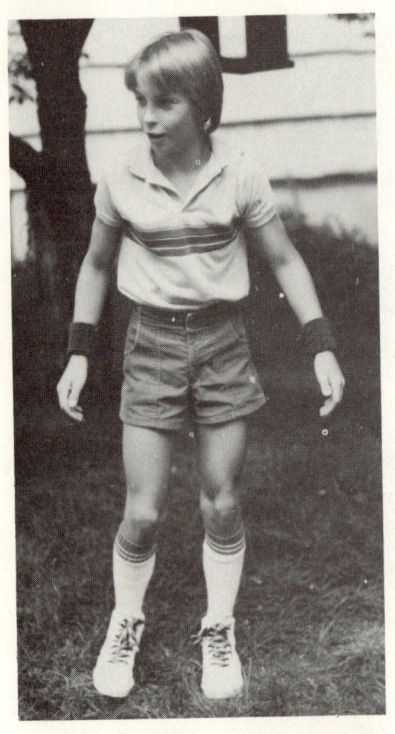

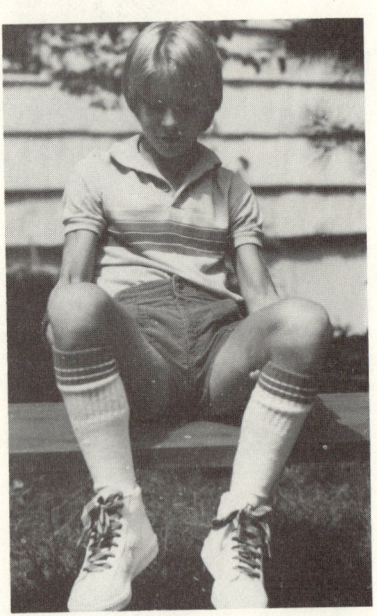

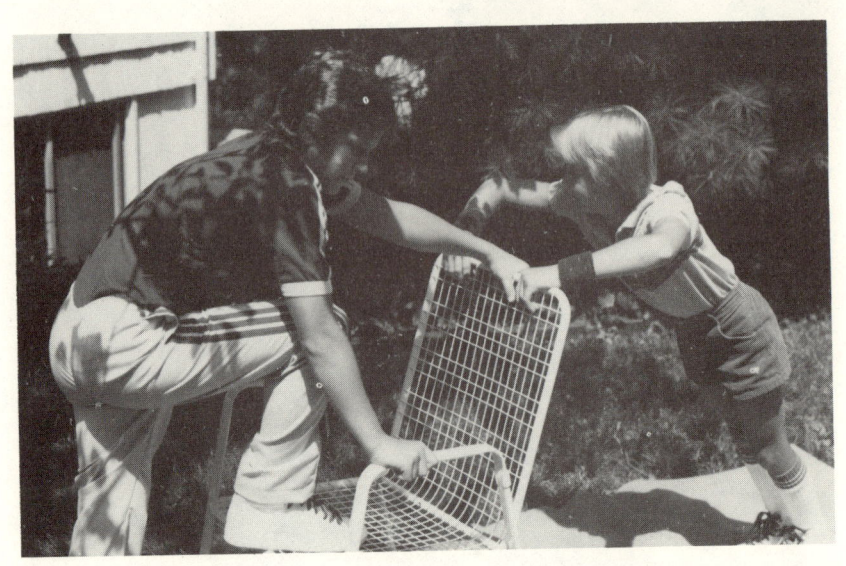

Walk in place for 2 minutes.

Push against a wall or have someone hold a chair and push against the back for 10 seconds. Relax for 5 and repeat again for 10 seconds.

This is a good relaxation exercise. Open eyes wide and close tightly 5 times and open hands wide and close tightly 5 times.

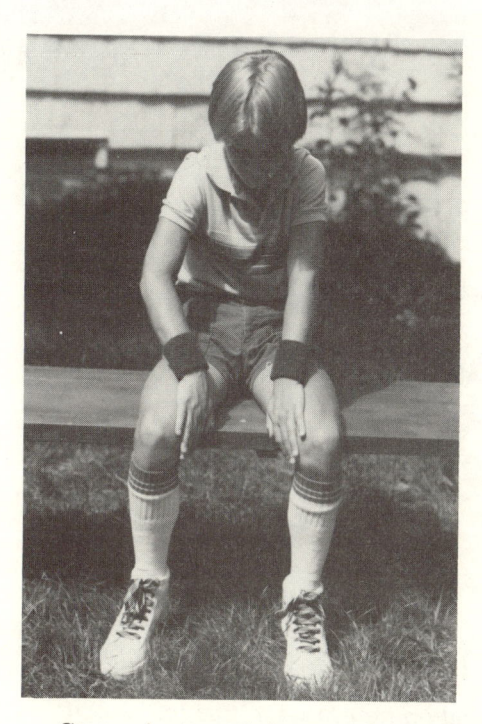

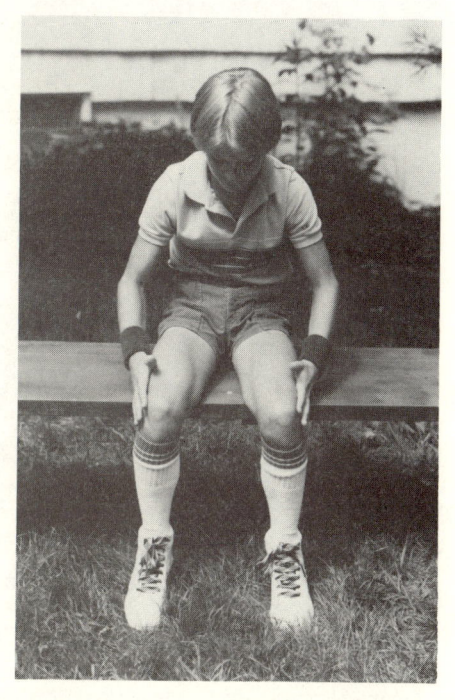

Sit in chair with knees about eight inches apart and lean forward, placing each palm on the outside of the corresponding knee. Push in with the arms while trying to keep the legs spread apart for the count of 5. Then place each palm on the inside of the corresponding knee and try to push the legs apart with the arms while resisting with the legs for the count of five.

Run in circles or figure eights for 1 minute without stopping.

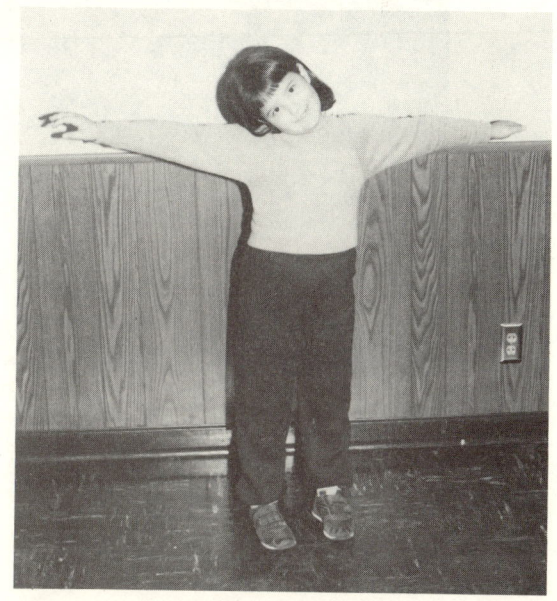

Swing arms side to side 20 times.

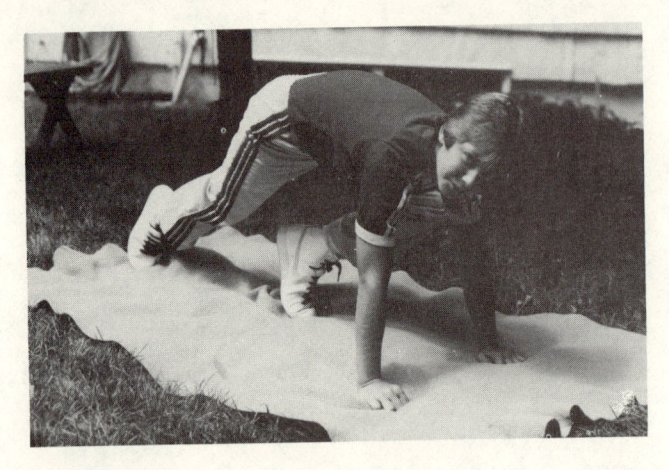

Squat with hands on floor, left leg extended to rear and right knee inside right elbow like a mountain climber. Reverse position of feet simultaneously. Again reverse positioning of feet, returning to starting position. Do 4 times.

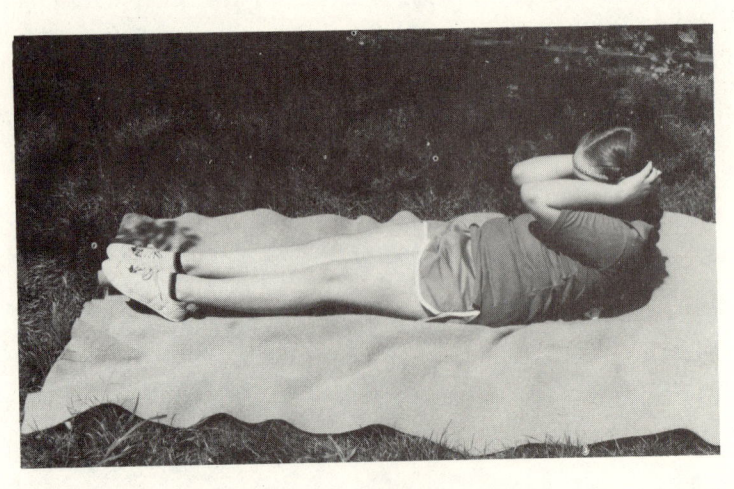

Lie on back, bend knees and interlace hands behind head. Tuck chin into chest and slowly curl forward until shoulders are about 10 inches off the floor, hold position for count of three. Return slowly to starting position. Repeat 5 times.

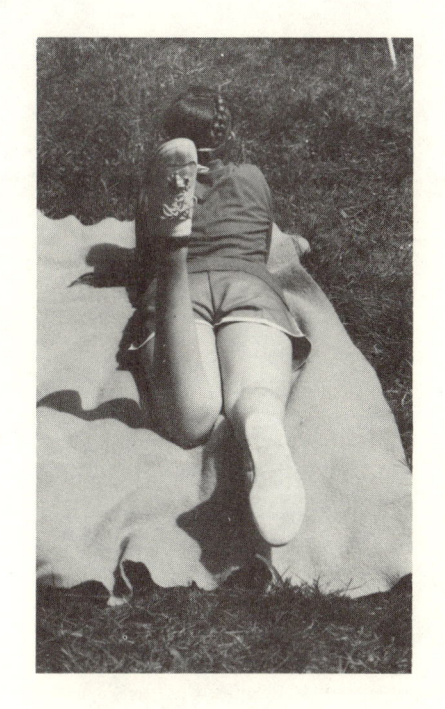

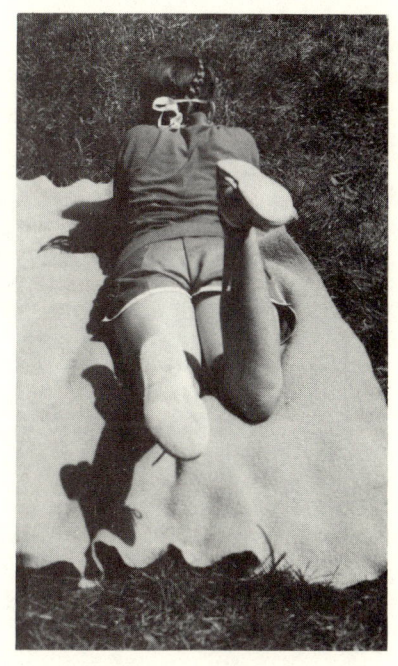

Lie on stomach and flutter legs as fast as possible for the count of 40.

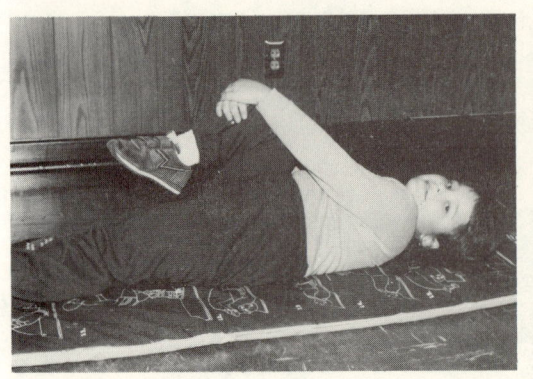

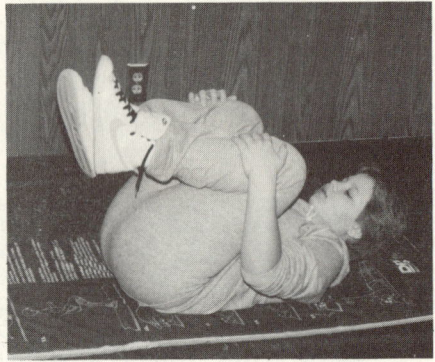

Lie on back, bring right knee to chest and grab it just below the knee and pull your knee slowly towards your chest. Hold stretched position for 5 seconds and repeat with the opposite leg. Do 5 times.

Lie on back and bring both knees to your chest. Grab each leg below the knee and pull both knees slowly towards your shoulder. Hold this stretch for 5 seconds and repeat 5 times.

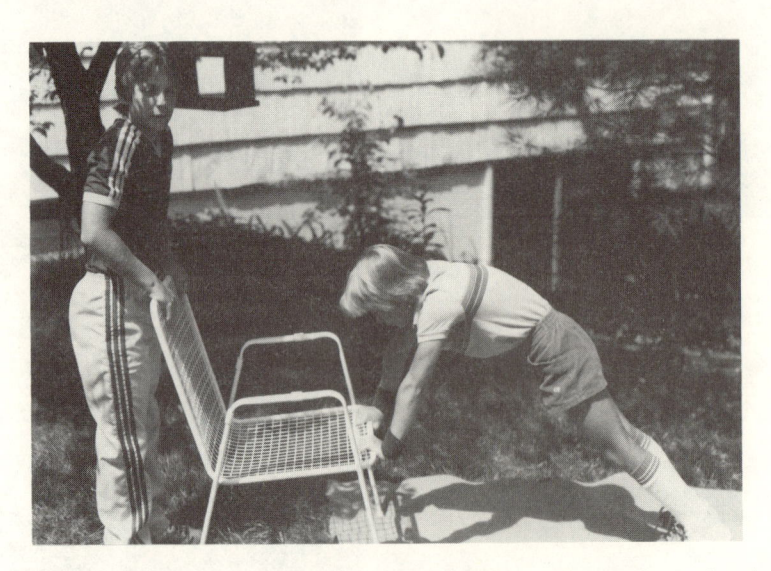

Place hands about shoulder width apart on front edge of a bed, sturdy chair or bench. Move feet backward until legs and back are in a straight line and your body weight is being supported only by your feet and your hands. Keep head up, bend arms at elbows and lower your body until chest touches front edge of bed. Push up, straightening arms until you have returned to starting position. Parent or a partner should spot for safety.

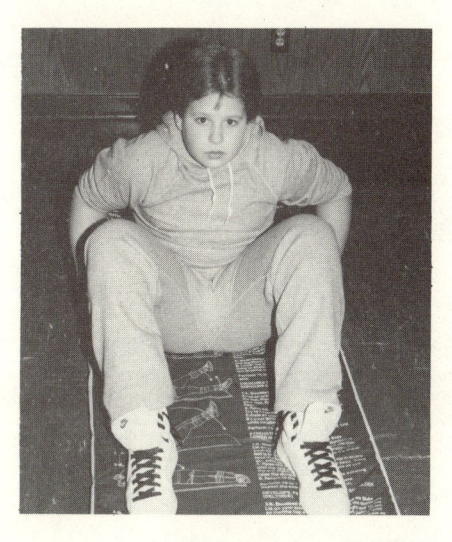

Some children cannot perform a sit-up because of their body weight and weak stomach muscles. To be able to get strong enough to perform a sit-up, they have to go through a full range of movements to strengthen stomach muscles. To start, they should first grab the pants on the side of their legs and use their arm muscles to assist them in doing sit-ups. After they work up to the point of doing 30 a day, they can start doing 5 sit-ups with the arms extended in front of them. When they reach 30, they can graduate to placing their arms across their chest. Again, they go back to 5 and build up to 30. Then they can put their hands behind their head in a conventional sit-up position, knees bent, feet flat on the floor. Starting at 5 and working up to 30, they can, if they really get good, put a telephone book behind their heads and perform the sit-ups to strengthen stomach muscles even more.

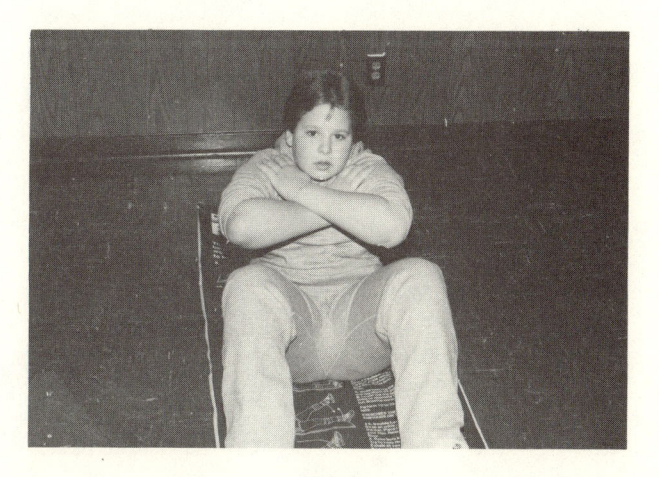

THIN KIDS

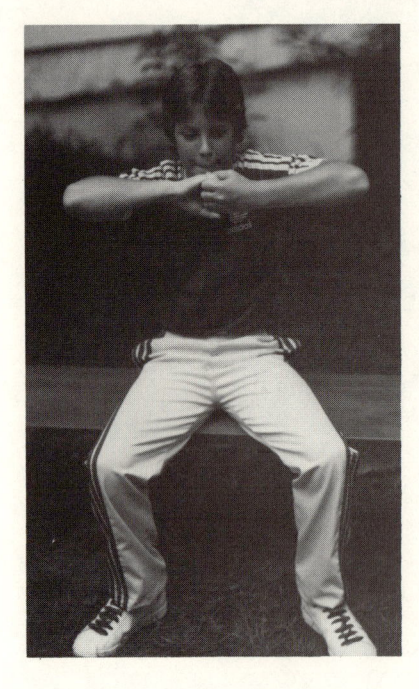

Grab your fingers with one thumb up and one thumb down and pull as hard as you can. Count to 10 and relax, repeat 5 times.

Run in place as fast as you can for 30 seconds.

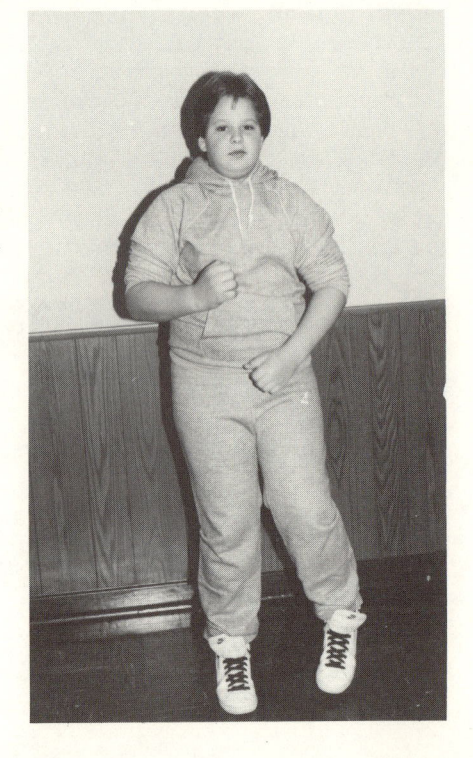

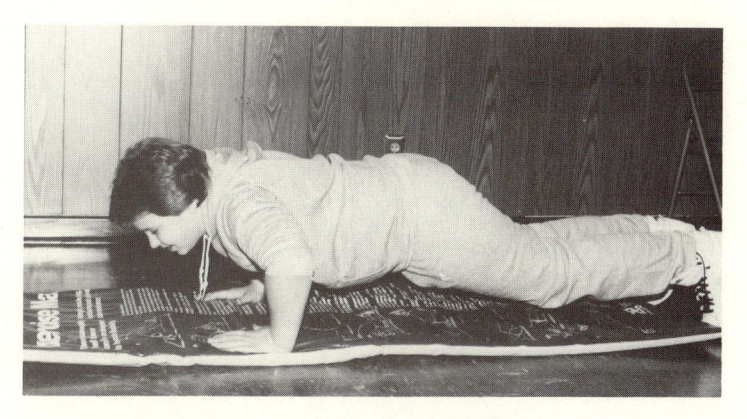

Lie on the floor in a prone position supporting yourself on your hands and toes. Push yourself off the floor and then lower yourself down. Try to keep your back straight and your stomach firm. Repeat 5 times.

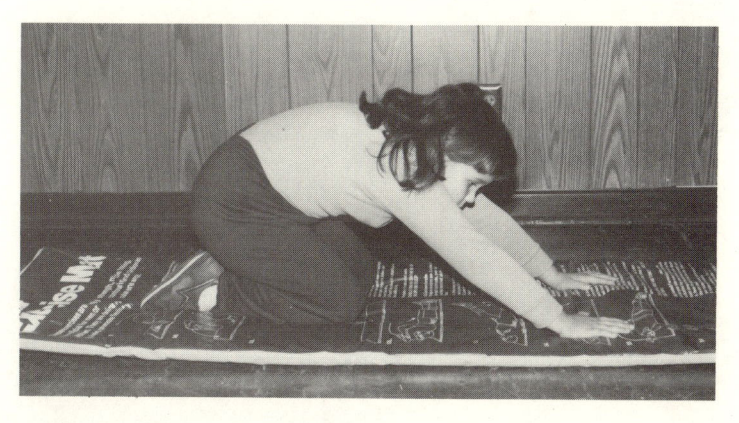

Start in the kneeling position with your knees 3 to 4 inches apart directly under your hips, and your arms directly under your shoulders. Swing your trunk forward over your shoulders, bend your elbows and lower your chest to the floor. Then, extend your arms forward, lower your head and raise your buttocks as high as you can by arching your back. Hold in this position for 5 seconds, then relax and repeat for a total of 5 repetitions.

THIN KIDS

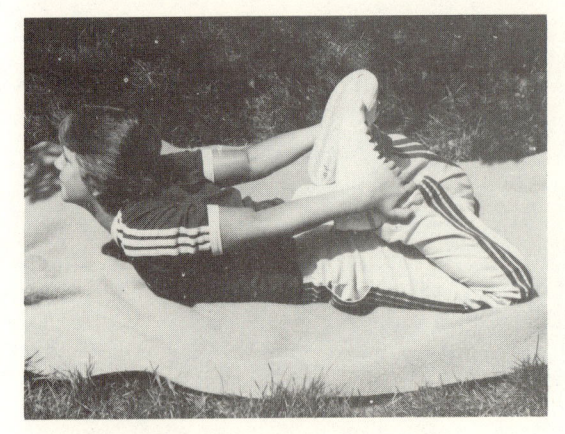

Lie flat on stomach, reach back and grab ankles, arching back and slowly pulling head up as high as possible. Hold this position for 5 seconds, then relax and repeat 3 times.

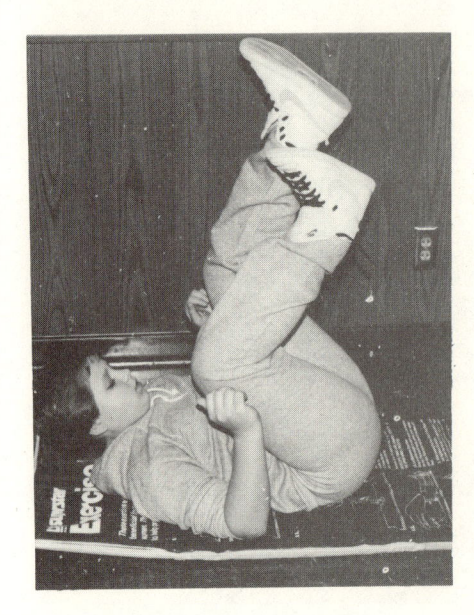

Lie on back and do bicycling in the air for 30 seconds.

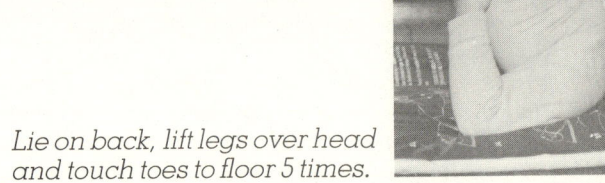

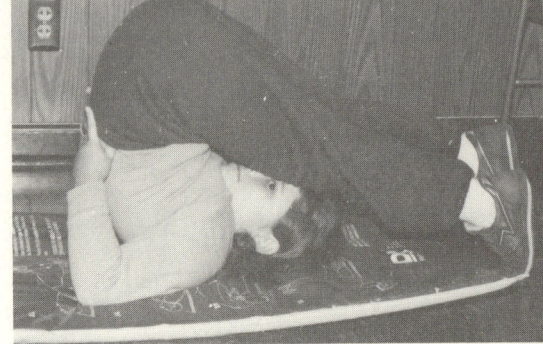

Lie on back, lift legs over head and touch toes to floor 5 times.

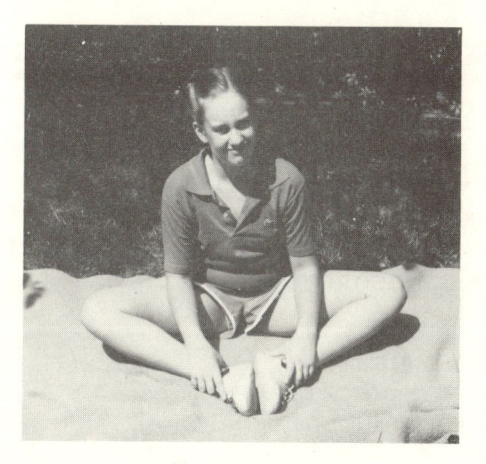

Sit on floor with soles of feet touching and knees pointing outward. Slowly push down on your knees, while gradually attempting to push them to the floor. Hold in stretched position for 5 seconds, relax and repeat 3 times.

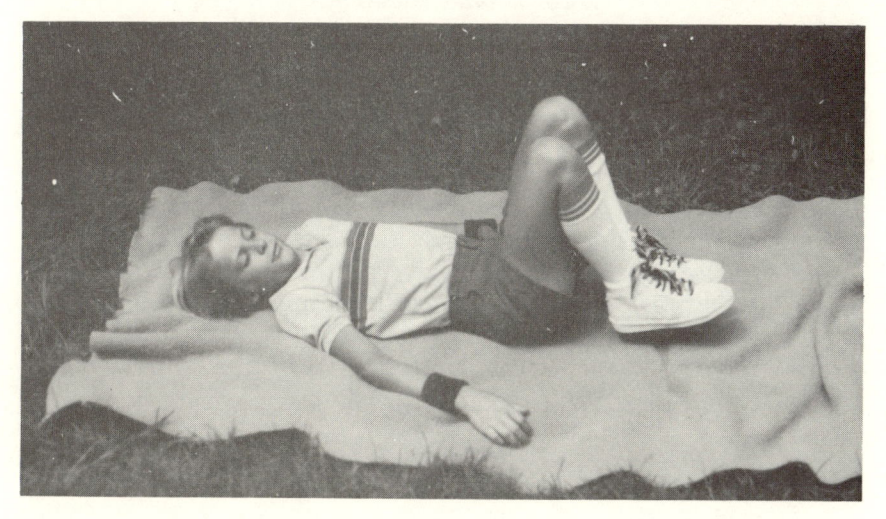

Lie on back and tense and relax all muscles 10 times.

Congratulations. You have completed your first set of 39 different exercises. Do the same next time or add repetitions.

NON-SPORT BUT USEFUL EXERCISES

Instead of eating a tangerine, have your child balance it on his head. Did you ever try walking a line balancing a book on your head without hands? Balancing objects on the head helps the sense of balance and improves coordination.

Here are some more physical activities that will be good for you as well as healthy for your child. Have your youngster:

- scrub the floors.
- clean out the garage.
- paint walls, outdoor furniture, etc.
- wash and wax the car.
- garden.
- ride a bike or walk on errands.

TIME TO EXERCISE

When a child first gets up, it is a good habit to do some stretching exercises and, of course, before any participation in sports or vigorous activity a youngster should stretch. No time of day is best for exercising. It is a matter of individual preference. Some children find it helps them sleep and some claim exercise helps them wake up. Strength promoting exercises are best done every other day or three times a week. The exercises aimed at increasing endurance should be done five or six times weekly and conditioning exercises should be done daily. Of course, those exercises which help parents—such as walking the dog and riding a bike for errands—should be done upon request.

CHAPTER VIII

THE THIN KIDS STRESS RELIEVERS

Believe it or not, children have many stresses, just as adults do. The tension may be caused by having trouble with homework, worry about taking a test, or not being asked to a dance, but the physical consequences are the same.

If your child can learn to relax, she will not only be able to respond better to a food program but to many areas of life and for a lifetime. Most stress response habits—including using food to ease tension—begin in youth.

Any technique that works will do. Here are two we use with a great deal of success in our Thin Kids Program. You can read the text while your child performs the actions or record the instructions on tape so that your child can perform the exercises anytime he chooses. Incidentally these relaxation techniques are good for all members of the family.

BASIC RELAXATION EXERCISE

- Get comfortable in a chair and then close your eyes.
- Tighten your leg and feet muscles. Now relax them and feel how relaxed your legs are.
- Tighten your stomach muscles. Make them really tight. Now relax your stomach muscles. Make them as relaxed as your legs all the way down to your feet.

Name _____   **PHYSICAL**

	Monday	Tuesday	Wednesday
7:00 8:00			
8:00 9:00			
9:00 10:00			
10:00 11:00			
11:00 12:00			
12:00 1:00			
1:00 2:00			
2:00 3:00			
3:00 4:00			
4:00 5:00			
5:00 6:00			
6:00 7:00			
7:00 8:00			
8:00 9:00			
9:00 10:00			

ACTIVITIES   Date _____

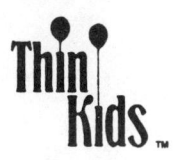

Thin Kids™

Thursday	Friday	Saturday	Sunday

- Keeping your eyes closed, stretch out your arms and make a very tight fist. As tight as possible, really gripping. Now relax your arms. See how relaxed your arms and your stomach and your legs and your feet are.
- Now slowly rock your head from side to side. This relaxes the neck muscles. Go very slowly, side to side. Now stop.
- Wrinkle up your face. Now relax your face.
- Press your tongue up against the roof of your mouth. Now relax your tongue. That helps your insides to relax.
- Feel how relaxed your face and your arms and your stomach and your legs are . . . all the way down to your toes.
- Now take a deep breath and then let it out very slowly, keeping all your muscles relaxed.
- You should feel relaxed all the way down to your feet.
- Now picture yourself in your favorite spot—under the sky, by the ocean, in the woods. See yourself there.
- At the same time, be silent for about two minutes and then count to five and open your eyes.

RAG DOLL RELAXER

The second method of relaxation—of course you can have your child do both—is a lot of fun. We call it The Rag Doll Relaxer.

1. Lie on the floor with a small pillow under your head. Your knees should be slightly bent. Put one hand on your stomach and one hand on your chest. Draw deep breaths into your abdomen and feel it rise. Your chest should hardly move at all. Belly-breathe without your chest moving and, as you exhale through your nose, try to say "cheese." Do this exercise five times. Then take a deep breath, as deep as you can, and exhale saying, "ha-a-a-a." Your jaw and tongue and mouth should be relaxed. Do this five times.

Hold your breath for the count of thirty. Then sigh,

deeply, letting all the air out of your lungs. Permit the air to return to your lungs naturally. Do this five times.

2. Stand with your knees slightly bent but not locked. Many tense people tend to lock their knees, which immobilizes the whole body. Take a position with your feet about eight inches apart and bend your knees so that the weight of your body is in balance between the heels and the balls of your feet. The rest of your body should be in a straight line with your arms hanging loosely at your side. Let your belly hang out. Do not force it out but do not hold it in. Belly-breathe. Your back should be straight but not rigid and your pelvis should be relaxed. Hold this position for the count of one hundred.

3. Stand up or sit up straight and look at the ceiling or sky. Smile and then blow an imaginary bubble high into the air. Repeat your smile and bubble blowing five times. This exercise loosens the neck, shoulder, and facial muscles tightened during tension.

4. Stand or sit and extend your arms straight out from your shoulders. Then swing both arms around yourself in a hug, and then extend them out again. Alternate putting your right arm over your left in the hug and then your left arm over your right. Do this with wild abandon ten times.

Your child should now be relaxed. Why not give her a hug?

PART 3
FACING FACTS ABOUT FOOD

CHAPTER IX

NUTRITION: WHAT EVERY THIN KID SHOULD KNOW

Now you and your child should be ready to embark on the Thin Kids food program. The first thing that should be clear is that everyone is on a diet. Some diets are high in calories and fats and some are calorie controlled and nutritious, as is the ten week plan.

As we have pointed out through the book, one of the major keys to making a food program work is to convince the child that he or she has control over the food they eat.

You can explain to your child that each of the broad food groups included in the Thin Kids food plan has a special job to do in fueling his engine and keep her body in tip top shape. You can ask your child to answer the quiz on page 90 and then go over the answers together.

What could be more interesting than understanding the fuel we put in our bodies to keep them moving and in good condition? Whatever your child's age, he can understand a great deal about nutrition.

If your child is too young to read food labels, read them to her and discuss the various desirable and undesirable ingredients.

The plan is three meals a day for ten weeks. Many overweight youngsters skip breakfast. Emphasize the necessity of having three meals a day to keep the engine running smoothly. He would not fill the car up with gas one time and then try to run it on empty another.

The program is designed to include from 1,550 to 1,850 calories per day, every day. To have a well-balanced, nutritious, satisfying program, every day's menu must include:

> Three servings of fruit,
> Three servings of milk,
> Eight ounces of protein,
> Three servings of bread,
> Three servings of fat,
> And the anytime foods.
> (See the list on page 205 of the various food groups.)

The foods in the milk group are a leading source of calcium, which is essential for the development of bones and teeth. Milk also contains high quality protein and is an excellent source of riboflavin, other vitamins, minerals, carbohydrates, and fat. Milk products such as cheese and ice cream supply these nutrients but in varied amounts. Whole milk normally contains very small amounts of vitamin D, but milk to which vitamin D has been added becomes a major source of this nutrient. We have low fat milk and ice cream products on our program, which retain the nutrients except the fat, and thus are better for children with weight problems.

The foods in the meat group are important for the amount and quality of the protein they provide. Protein is important mainly as a tissue builder. It is a part of muscle, organs, blood, skin, hair, and other living tissues. Dried beans, peas, and nuts also supply protein but not of the same quality of meat and milk. Beside protein, meats provide iron, thiamine, riboflavin, and niacin.

Vegetables and fruits are valuable because of the vitamins and minerals they contain. Vitamin A is very important for the growth and development in children of normal vision and for a healthy skin. Another important vitamin is ascorbic acid or vitamin C, which is essential for healthy gums and body tissues.

Breads and cereals—whole grain, enriched, restored—

NUTRITION

furnish worthwhile amounts of thiamine, iron, niacin, protein, and food energy.

All the foods listed in our program are readily available at your supermarket. Our program is nutritionally balanced but you may want to talk to your child's physician about supplementary vitamins.

As we have said over and over again, we emphasize the child's own control over the menu. If your youngster hates peas, for example, he can substitute any vegetable. If he would rather have hamburgers instead of lamb chops, substitute one meat for the other. Your child can pick and choose among the suggested menus and the recipes, just so long as he or she has three proteins a day, three milks, three breads, three fruits and at least two vegetables.

Many children say that they hate some item, such as tomato juice. We ask them to try it again, since tastes do change. They may say they hate broccoli and we suggest they try it made another way and maybe then they will like it.

Don't force your child to try a new food. We do emphasize variety and sometimes, if you offer an incentive for trying something, such as a new magazine or talking fifteen minutes longer on the telephone, they may try it and like it.

It is not unusual for a child to live on a very limited menu. Freddie, for example, who was in a Thin Kids group, ate nothing but peanut butter and bread and milk and could not understand why he was so overweight. When we weaned him away from his limited diet, we suggested he make himself a tossed salad with whole peanuts mixed in. He liked that and began just eating that, but eventually he learned to balance his diet and lost twenty pounds.

Seeing children like Freddie go through the ten week program and not only lose weight but develop healthy habits that will last throughout their lives is very rewarding. We are sure that if you and your child follow The Thin Kids Program for ten weeks, you will see a great difference.

The diet is portion-controlled, well-balanced nutritionally, and there is enough choice to please any kid—even Freddie.

The following is a suggested meal plan:

Breakfast:

One ounce of protein, such as an egg or a half cup of cottage cheese
One bread, such as two-thirds of a cup of cereal or a pocket pita
One milk, such as a glass of low fat milk or a cup of low calorie yogurt
One fruit, such as an orange or half a grapefruit
One fat, such as a tablespoon of light margarine

Lunch:

Three ounces of protein, such as turkey or tuna
One bread, such as two thin breads or 3 bread sticks
A fruit, such as an apple or a pear or a cup of berries
A tablespoon of fat, such as light mayonnaise or two tablespoons of light salad dressing
One milk, such as a cup of low fat milk
Unlimited vegetables, such as carrot and celery sticks or salad

Snack:

Low calorie ice cream pop; or a cup of broth with two crackers; or a cup of low calorie yogurt; or fruit pop; or popcorn

Dinner:

Four ounces of protein such as broiled fish, turkey, hamburger, or lamb
One bread, such as a baked or broiled potato or half cup of pasta or rice
Green vegetable such as broccoli, string beans or spinach
Large salad, including all favorite vegetables
One fat, such as a tablespoon of light margarine or two tablespoons of light salad dressing.
Optional food, such as a cup of V-8 or tomato juice and/or a cup of broth.
Fruit for dessert could be saved for a snack such as frozen grapes, baked apple, fruit cup, or fresh fruit

ALWAYS, ALWAYS . . .

- Always weigh and measure your foods and drinks
- Always trim-off extra fat from meat
- Always remove chicken skin after cooking
- Always drink a lot of water
- Always eat at least three meals a day
- Always help yourself to plenty of vegetables
- Always plan alternative activities for problem eating times
- Always have tuna packed in water
- Always have fruit packed in natural juice
- Always read food labels so that you can make wise choices
- Always restrict artificial sweeteners, including diet drinks
- Always eat a well-balanced diet

CHAPTER X

QUIZ: HOW MUCH HAVE YOU LEARNED ABOUT FOOD?

QUIZ—NUTRITION QUESTIONS TO ASK YOUR CHILD AND TO DISCUSS

What are the four food groups?

Answer: Milk and dairy products, meats, breads and grains, fruits and vegetables. A well-balanced meal should include at least one serving of each.

What are calories?

Answer: Actually a calorie is the amount of heat required to raise the temperature of one gram of water from 14.5 to 15.5 degrees centigrade at atmospheric pressure. But it is usually used as a measure of the energy value of food as well as the energy the human body uses for activities and for maintaining body processes.

Why count calories?

Answer: The balance of calories—energy in the food—you eat versus the energy—the calories—that you use up in a day can gauge how much weight a body can lose or gain. To gain a pound you must eat 3,500 more calories than you use up.

HOW MUCH HAVE YOU LEARNED?

Why will an empty calorie stimulate your appetite?

Answer: An empty calorie is a refined carbohydrate, like table sugar. It goes right into the blood stream, has little nutritive value, and raises blood sugar levels and then drops them. It stimulates the appetite and also reminds kids of the taste of sweets such as candy and cakes.

What are some of the various types (or names) of sugars?

Answer: Different types of sugars include: Dextrose, sucrose, fructose, lactose, maltose, corn syrup, honey, molasses, brown sugar, powdered sugar.

Why should you be careful of fats?

Answer: Because fat has twice as many calories per teaspoonful as protein and other food sources.

What is cholesterol?

Answer: Cholesterol is waxy fat that occurs in all animal tissues and in egg yolk and blood. It is important in the metabolism but has been implicated as contributing to hardening of the arteries and subsequently to heart attacks. Cholesterol is a saturated fat.

What is a saturated fat?

Answer: Saturated fats are usually solid at room temperature. Most animals fats are saturated but butterfat, coconut oil, and peanut oil are high in saturated fats. Eating too much of the saturated fats, such as cholesterol, is thought to contribute to heart disease and blood vessel disease.

What is an unsaturated fat?

Answer: Unsaturated fats are usually liquid at room temperature. Vegetable oils and fish oils most frequently contain unsaturated fats, which are supposed to be less likely to cause clogging of the arteries.

What do doctors mean when they say something is a risk factor?

Answer: Risk factors are associated with an increased risk of developing heart disease. These characteristics include high blood pressure, elevated blood cholesterol [and other fats], [cigarette smoking], obesity, diabetes, and a family history of heart disease. Discuss this with your kid, but do not frighten her. Just explain that she has plenty of time to prevent problems later in life by paying attention to what she is eating now.

Why should you eat fiber?

Answer: Fibers in fruits and vegetables move through the intestinal tract like a sponge and soak up and remove foreign substances that may be bad for you. They also help relieve constipation and they make you feel full so that you are not very hungry. Since you cannot digest fibers, they have no calories.

Which makes you fuller, a glass of orange juice or an orange?

Answer: Most kids have found that eating the orange is more filling, because it is higher in fiber and takes longer to eat and you chew it. Do an experiment for yourself. Cut half an orange and have half a glass of orange juice. The orange is more satisfying psychologically, and its fiber is an added benefit.

Why do we need fruit?

Answer: Fruit is nature's candy. Fruits have vitamins and fibers and are a good source of energy. The sugar in them is easily digested by the body.

Why eat vegetables?

Answer: Vegetables are high in fiber, low in calories, and loaded with vitamins. They are good to use for snacks rather than high calorie candy bars and chips.

HOW MUCH HAVE YOU LEARNED?

What does product labeling tell us?

Answer: The ingredients in the food are listed in descending order. That is, the largest ingredient is listed first. It also tells us the nutritional value of food—the fat, protein, and vitamins—and how much a serving is. You do not really know what you are eating until you read the labels.

What is another name for salt?

Answer: Sodium. Look at labels and see how much sodium is in a product. We often get too much and it can raise blood pressure and make us retain fluids. Our foods have enough salt naturally without adding table salt.

Why is it important to drink a lot of water?

Answer: Water maintains body function, flushes out the body, and dampens the appetite. It also helps keep the skin in good condition.

Why do we need vitamins?

Answer: Because vitamins are literally vital to a healthy living organism.

What does vitamin A do?

Answer: Vitamin A is essential for growth and vision, and aids in combating infection. It is also good for the skin. Good sources of it are fruits and vegetables, dairy products, cod liver oil, kidney, liver, and oysters.

What are the B vitamins?

Answer: The vitamin B complex includes the following.
Thiamine, or vitamin B-1, is found in meats and vegetables, whole grains, and in brewers' yeast. It is good for the teeth and gums, promotes growth, aids in carbohydrate metabolism, and stimulates the appetite.
Riboflavin, known as vitamin B-2, is found in the same

foods as thiamine. Riboflavin deficiency results in a burning of the eyes, lips, tongue, and may cause loss of hair.

Niacin is found in foods rich in riboflavin. Deficiency of niacin results in pellagra, a disease that causes reddening of parts of the body, stomach upsets and nerve problems.

Pyridoxine, vitamin B-6, is found in egg yolk, wheat germ, and yeast. It is necessary to digest fats and to have healthy blood.

Vitamin B-12 is used in the treatment of certain blood disorders. It is found in the liver.

What does vitamin C do?

Answer: Also called ascorbic acid, it is found in all types of vegetables and fruits, especially citrus fruits. It is needed to keep the teeth, gums, and joints healthy and to hold the body together. There is some research that says vitamin C can prevent colds and other infections, but not everyone agrees.

Why do we need vitamin D?

Answer: This vitamin aids in the development of bones and teeth. Deficiency causes crooked, weak bones in children. Sources include fruits and vegetables, fortified dairy products, cod liver oil, liver, kidneys, and oysters.

What is vitamin E good for?

Answer: This vitamin protects the blood against damage and is now believed to play a role in disease prevention, including certain cancers. But scientists are still not sure of all its functions. It can be found in green vegetables and wheat germ oil.

Did you ever hear of vitamin K?

Answer: It is manufactured in the intestines, but if we need more of it, we usually get a synthetic K made in the laboratory. This vitamin helps the blood to clot and prevent hemorrhaging.

Why do we need calcium?

Answer: We need calcium for strong bones, teeth, muscles and for nerve function. Calcium can be found in dairy products, nuts, legumes, sardines, oysters, soy beans, wheat germ, cabbage, and turnip greens.

Will iron make us strong?

Answer: Iron is essential for red blood cell manufacture and without it, we would be very weak. It can be found in green leafy vegetables, meat, brewers' yeast, wheat germ, eggs, seeds, almonds, parsley, prunes, and raisins.

What is zinc for?

Answer: Zinc is essential for growth, good skin, and wound healing.

Do we need potassium?

Answer: We certainly do. It is necessary for proper cell function and our muscles would be weak without it. Nuts, seeds, and fruits are high in potassium.

Why is it important to eat three meals a day?

Answer: Breakfast is literally that—breaking the fast of the night. You have not eaten for at least twelve hours. Breakfast gives you energy to start the day. If you skip breakfast, then you will be hungrier at lunch and eat more than the 300–400 calories you skipped during breakfast. If you skip lunch, you will build up a tremendous hunger after school and will probably eat anything that is available, including high calorie foods. A well-balanced dinner makes you feel full so that you will not be looking for snacks all evening.

CHAPTER XI

HINTS AND SUGGESTIONS FROM MINDY, LOU, AND SOME THIN KIDS

Obtain medical advice before putting a child on a diet. Your child should have a physical examination since there are medical conditions that may cause obesity, and even a healthy child should have dietary recommendations, because proper nutrition is vital to growth.

Make sure your child does not skip meals. Hunger builds; blood sugar drops, and your child will eat junk foods or overeat at a meal.

Help your child plan meals and snacks each day that are nutritious and calorie controlled. The more in charge children feel of their own diets, the more cooperative they will be. Take your child to the supermarket and let the youngster select nutritious, calorie controlled foods for the entire family by reading labels.

Make plans for your personal problem times—have a list of substitute activities ready to do.

Set a time each day during which you and your child will sit down and discuss how the day went—the problems and the successes.

HINTS AND SUGGESTIONS

If your child tells you a problem during your special discussion time, instead of emphasizing the failure, help her make it into a positive learning experience. Brainstorm with your child about making those problems easier to handle next time.

Set up some kind of support system within the family. Sisters and brothers can be detrimental or supportive. You have got to get them to be the latter.

Keep the food plan and the diary sheet attached to the refrigerator with a magnet. Have your child fill it in after every meal and snack.

Put signs on the refrigerator and pantry saying "Is this food worth it?"

Realize how difficult it is for a young person to cope with the temptation of boxes of cookies in the house. Or how much control is required to select less fattening food if the rest of the family is enjoying it.

Don't use dessert to discipline your child.

Don't put all the food on the table at once—that encourages second helpings.

Does Sunday dinner at a restaurant have to be a big outting?

Colorful food combinations are more fun and more appetizing for children. Try oranges, yellows, greens, and reds.

Let your youngster use cookie cutters to make fun sandwiches.

Use your imagination. A piece of melon can become a sail boat and a cup of cottage cheese can have a clown's face, with some pimentos and raisins.

Never force a child to eat.

Set a good example. The eating habits of parents and older siblings greatly influence a child's food behavior.

Four to six small meals a day instead of three may make weight control easier for your child.

Hints from Thin Kids Themselves and Their Parents

"Take a hot dog or hamburger roll and slice it in half so that you have half a top and half a bottom. Then put your hamburger or hot dog in there and you can still enjoy the bun but with less calories." Arnold, 7 years old

"Take the skin off the chicken, squeeze half a lemon over it, sprinkle garlic powder on it and a teaspoon of soy sauce and cook it on your backyard barbecue." Lynn, 14 years old

"Just tell yourself when you are tempted how good you will feel after you lose weight and how people will envy your willpower. Think how good you will look and feel in your clothes, mostly in a bathing suit, and think of someone you want to impress." Kelly, 16 years old

"Put an ice pop stick in a banana and freeze the banana. It tastes just like ice cream." Bobby, 9 years old

"When other people are eating something you would like to eat and shouldn't, walk away." Petie, 8 years old

"On my trip it was very hard for me to get in all of my milks. The fruits were kind of easy but the bread was kind of hard. At dinner the rolls were very tempting, but I'm so proud of myself . . . I didn't eat them! I tried many things but only had a little taste of each one. I did a lot of walking on this trip. By the end of the day I was tired." Marla, 12 years old

"When I had the urge to eat I would take a piece of fruit and a glass of water and do my exercises, and that would fill me up." Lizzie, 7 years old

"Most children were calling me names concerning my weight. I was growing out of clothes very quickly. Now everybody notices that I have lost weight. My former sizes of clothing are becoming loose." Pam, 14 years old

"I must admit that as well as I know my child, I didn't realize how determined she was. She didn't have any difficulty staying on the program. I believe the main reason for this was planning. Whether a holiday, birthday, or tomorrow's lunch, the day before she would decide what she would have We worked together on this and had no problems. My

HINTS AND SUGGESTIONS

daughter is the same bright, lovable, terrific child, but now her energy level and involvement in sports, as well as social situations, is boundless. If Jannie passes mirrors, she smiles into them. That's success." The mother of 13-year-old Jannie

"Sugarless bubble gum is great when you are tempted."

Jeff, 10 years old

"She is more alert and raises her hand to be called on and she volunteers to do things for the teacher. Her self-image did change. She goes up to kids and makes friends. She's confident in herself. You have to work hard with your child and don't get discouraged because it makes it harder for them. We would always praise her and say that she was doing a great job. We gave her something to look forward to, like rewarding her when she lost a certain amount of weight. We bought her all new summer clothes and she loved that very much." The mother of 10-year-old Laura

"Throwing snowballs is great exercise and a lot of fun."

Joseph, 8 years old

PART 4
THE THIN KIDS FOOD PLAN

CHAPTER XII:

TEN WEEKS OF COMPLETE THIN KIDS MENUS

On the following pages you'll find ten full weeks of easy and delicious Thin Kids meals that your whole family will enjoy. But before you begin you should make yourself familiar with the important items listed below. They all play an important part in making your new way of eating fun, easy, and effective.

<u>Cooking Utensils</u>
  Diet scale (for weighing your food portions)
  Silverstone pan (for frying food with a minimum of fat)
  Non-stick cooking spray (for frying food with a minimum of calories)
  Air popcorn popper (for popping corn without excess oil or butter)
  Plastic wraps and containers (for wrapping pre-measured food portions and keeping them fresh in the refrigerator)
  Measuring cups and spoons (for exact measurements of food in recipes)

<u>Special Food Items</u>
  Rice cakes (Low calorie bread substitute; found in most supermarkets)
  Pocket pitas (Far-eastern flat, hollow bread—ideal for sandwiches)

Name _____ **FOOD**

	Sunday	Monday	Tuesday
B R E A K F A S T	Pocket pita 1 egg 1 oz. cheese ½ grapefruit 1 C. low fat milk	⅔ C. cereal 1 C. low fat milk 1 egg 1 tbsp. lgt. marg.	1 egg 1 thin bread 1 C. low fat milk ½ cantaloupe
L U N C H	½ Eng. muffin 3 oz. cheese 2 tbsp. sauce Sautéed veg. 1 pear 1 C. low fat milk	3 oz. chicken 1 pocket pita 1 apple 6 oz. tom. juice Carrot & celery sticks	Chef Salad: 1 oz. turkey 1 oz. roast beef 1 oz. cheese salad 2 tbsp. low-cal salad dress. 2 crackers 1 C. low fat milk
D I N N E R	4 oz. chicken ½ C. noodles Large salad ½ C. veg. 1 tbsp. lgt. marg. 2 tbsp. low-cal salad dress. 1 C. whipped yogurt 6 oz. tom. juice	4 oz. meat loaf Baked potato 1 tbsp. lgt. marg. Large salad 2 tbsp. low-cal salad dress. Vegetables 1 C. low-cal yogurt	6 cooked shrimp 3 oz. meat ball ½ C. pasta ½ C. tom. sauce Salad 1 C. fruit bowl
S N A C K S	Thin Kids Juice pop ½ C. berries	½ C. raw cauliflower 6 oz. orange juice ½ C. fruit salad	1 plum 1½ C. popped popcorn 1 tbsp. lgt. marg.

Include Time

INTAKE   Date _____

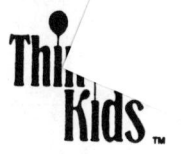

Thin Kids™

Wednesday	Thursday	Friday	Saturday
1 rice cake 1 tbsp. peanut butter 1 C. low-cal yogurt 1 orange	⅔ C. cereal 1 C. low fat milk 2 oz. ricotta cheese ½ C. strawberries	1 thin bread 1 oz. cheese 1 orange ½ C. low fat milk	½ C. cottage cheese 1 C. low fat milk 1 C. strawberries Vanilla
3 oz. chicken Tossed salad 1½ breadsticks 2 tbsp. low-cal salad dress. 1 apple 1 C. low fat milk 1½ C. popped popcorn	3 oz. tuna 1 tbsp. lgt. mayo 3 tbsp. chooped celery 1 pocket pita Lettuce & tomato 1 orange 1 C. low fat milk	3 oz. turkey roll 1 pocket pita 1 tbsp lgt. mayo 1 C. low fat milk Salad 2 tbsp. low-cal salad dress.	3 tbsp. peanut butter 1 tbsp. low-sugar jelly 2 thin breads Raw vegetable 1 small banana
4 oz. lamb patty ½ C. wide noodles 1 tbsp. lgt. marg. Broccoli spears Salad 2 tbsp. low-cal salad dress. 1 low-cal ice cream pop	4 oz. turkey Baked potato Vegetables 1 tbsp. lgt. marg. Salad 2 tbsp. low-cal salad dress. ¼ cantaloupe	4 oz. broiled fish 1 tbsp. lgt. marg. ⅛ C. brd. crmbs. ½ C. rice 1 C. chicken broth Vegetables Salad 2 tbsp. low-cal salad dress.	4 oz. London broil 1 boiled potato 1 tbsp. lgt. marg. 1 cup vegetables Tossed salad 2 tbsp. low-cal salad dress. 1 baked apple
6 oz. tom. juice Celery sticks ½ C. fruit slices	½ C. peaches 1 C. low-cal yogurt Raw veggies	1 apple, sliced Low-calorie ice cream pop	1 C. low-calorie yogurt 3 C. popped popcorn 1 tbsp. lgt. marg.

Name _____ **FOOD**

	Sunday	Monday	Tuesday
BREAKFAST			
LUNCH			
DINNER			
SNACKS			

Include Time

INTAKE Date _____

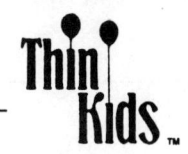

Thin Kids

Wednesday	Thursday	Friday	Saturday

Seltzer (Carbonated water—Buy brands marked "low-sodium")
Low calorie mayonnaise
Low calorie salad dressing
Light (low calorie) margarine
Low calorie yogurt
Low fat milk
Low calorie ice cream pops
Diet breadsticks
Vegetable juices
Herbs and Spices (Oregano, Garlic, Rosemary, Parsley, Paprika, etc., etc.)

<u>Food Intake Charts</u>

On the preceding pages you will find two samples of a Food Intake Chart. One has been filled in as an example and the other is for you to copy and fill out with your child each day. It is important to keep a daily record of all food eaten so that your child can see his progress and have an incentive to keep up the good work. Such a record also makes it easier for you to see the strong and weak areas of your child's diet and this will help you decide if he needs more protein or less carbohydrates, for example.

Now you are both ready to read and follow the Thin Kids Menus. Remember that it is important to eat three meals a day and the snacks provided. This helps to train the appetite and will make weight loss much easier. If you must make substitutions, try to keep them within the same calorie range, and remember all our advice about eating in restaurants and at parties.

Ready? It's up to you and your child now. Good luck!

WEEK ONE

DAY 1 — WEEK 1

	Calories	Total Calories
Breakfast:		
1 egg	85	
1 thin slice bread	40	
1 cup low calorie yogurt	150	
*Frozen Orange Smiles (p. 200)	70	
1 tbsp. light margarine	50	**395**
Lunch:		
3 ounces turkey	150	
1 pocket pita bread	80	
1 apple	75	
Carrot and celery sticks	35	
1 tbsp. light mayonnaise	50	
1 cup low fat milk	120	**510**
Snack:		
Low calorie ice cream pop	100	**100**
Dinner:		
*Thin Kids Fish Delight (p. 197)	380	
Large salad	50	
1 cup frozen string beans or broccoli	40	
1 small potato, baked	50	
1 tbsp. light margarine	50	
2 tbsp. low calorie salad dressing	50	**620**
Snack:		
*Thin Kids Ice Pops (p. 199)	90	**90**

*Recipe is given in recipe section.

Total Calories: 1,715

DAY 2 ▶ WEEK 1

	Calories	Total Calories
Breakfast:		
⅔ cup cereal	80	
1 cup low fat milk	120	
*Frozen Banana Treat (p. 200)	80	
½ cup cottage cheese	120	**400**
Lunch:		
*Toss The Log Salad (p. 191)	350	
1 pear	100	
1 cup low fat milk	120	**570**
Snack:		
1 cup chicken broth	50	
2 crackers	35	**85**
Dinner:		
*Burger Build-Up (p. 193)	400	
1 cup string beans	40	
1 tbsp. light margarine	50	
1 cup low calorie yogurt	150	**640**
Snack:		
*Frozen Grape Sensation (p. 200)	50	**50**

Total Calories: 1,745

DAY 3 — WEEK 1

	Calories	Total Calories
Breakfast:		
*Open Face Melted Cheese Supreme (p. 194)	150	
1 orange	70	
1 cup low fat milk	120	**340**
Lunch:		
3 ounces tuna	165	
1 tbsp. light mayonnaise	40	
Chopped celery	5	
Carrot sticks	25	
2 thin slices of bread	80	
1 apple	65	
1 cup low fat milk	120	**500**
Snack:		
1 cup low calorie yogurt	150	**150**
Dinner:		
4 ounces chicken	200	
1 cup chicken broth	50	
Large green salad	50	
1 cup green vegetable	40	
2 tbsp. low calorie dressing	25	
1 medium potato, baked	90	**455**
Snack:		
½ cup fruit cup	70	**70**

Total Calories: 1,515

DAY 4 — WEEK 1

	Calories	Total Calories
Breakfast:		
*Cottage Cheese Morning Danish (p. 183)	235	
1 cup low fat milk	120	**355**
Lunch:		
*Thin Kids Pizza (p. 196)	320	
½ cup fruit cup	70	
1 cup low fat milk	120	
Small green salad	35	
2 tbsp. low calorie salad dressing	25	**570**
Snack:		
Low calorie ice cream pop	100	**100**
Dinner		
*Chicken in the Pot (p. 196)	385	
Small green salad	50	
2 tbsp. low calorie salad dressing	25	**460**
Snack:		
*Apple Surprise (p. 199)	110	**110**

Total Calories: 1,595

MENUS

DAY 5 — WEEK 1

	Calories	Total Calories
Breakfast:		
1 egg	80	
⅔ cup cereal	80	
1 cup low fat milk	120	
½ cup peaches	50	
1 tbsp. light margarine	50	**380**
Lunch:		
3 oz. chicken (skinless)	150	
Lettuce and tomato	25	
1 orange	75	
1 small can V-8 or tomato juice	35	
1 cup chicken broth	50	
2 crackers	35	**370**
Snack:		
2 Thin Kids Ice Pops (6 oz. juice) (p. 199)	90	**90**
Dinner:		
1 serving *Meat Loaf Italiano (p. 195)	265	
½ cup pasta	100	
½ cup tomato sauce	50	
Small green salad	50	
2 tbsp. low calorie dressing	50	
1 cup low fat milk	120	
4 broccoli spears	40	
½ tbsp. light margarine	25	**700**
Snack:		
1 cup low calorie yogurt	150	**150**

Total Calories: 1,690

DAY 6 ▶ WEEK 1

	Calories	Total Calories
Breakfast:		
1 rice cake	35	
1 tbsp. peanut butter	105	
1 cup low calorie yogurt	150	
½ cup low fat milk	60	
½ cup grapefruit	45	**395**
Lunch:		
*Reverse Sandwiches (p. 193)	350	
1 cup low fat milk	120	
1 orange	70	
Raw vegetables	25	
1 tbsp. light mayonnaise	40	**605**
Snack:		
*Frozen Grape Sensation (p. 200)	50	**50**
*Thin Kids Fish Delight (p. 197)	315	
½ cup cauliflower	15	
Lettuce and tomato	25	
1 tbsp. low calorie dressing	25	
1 medium potato, baked	90	
1 cup chicken broth	50	**520**
Snack:		
*Thin Kids Ice Pop (p. 199)	100	
Carrot and celery sticks	25	
1 small sliced cucumber	20	**145**

Total Calories: 1,715

DAY 7 ▶ WEEK 1

	Calories	Total Calories
Breakfast:		
1 egg	80	
*Thin Kids Fruited Milk Shake (p. 186)	200	**280**
Lunch:		
1 pocket pita	80	
3 ounces chopped cooked chicken	120	
1 tbsp. light mayonnaise	40	
Chopped celery	10	
1 apple	70	
1 small can V-8 or tomato juice	35	**355**
Snack:		
1 cup low calorie yogurt	150	**150**
Dinner:		
4 ounces cooked shrimp	100	
4 ounces cooked veal burger	240	
½ cup cooked rice	100	
1 cup stewed tomato and zucchini	45	
1 cup green vegetables	40	
1 tbsp. light margarine	50	
Small green salad	50	
2 tbsp. low calorie dressing	50	**675**
Snack:		
½ cup low calorie ice cream	100	**100**

Total Calories: 1,560

WEEK TWO

DAY 1 ▶ WEEK 2

	Calories	Total Calories
Breakfast:		
⅔ cup cereal	80	
1 cup low fat milk	120	
1 egg scrambled	80	
1 tbsp. light margarine	50	**330**
Lunch:		
3 ounces sliced chicken	150	
1 pocket pita	80	
1 apple	70	
1 6 ounce can tomato juice	35	
Carrot and celery sticks	25	**360**
Snack:		
½ cup raw cauliflower	15	
6 ounces *Orange Slush (p. 186)	90	**105**
Dinner:		
1 serving *Meat Loaf Italiano (p. 195)	265	
1 medium potato, baked	90	
1 tbsp. light margarine	50	
Large salad	50	
2 tbsp. light salad dressing	25	
Large piece cauliflower	15	
2 broccoli spears	20	
1 cup low calorie yogurt	150	**665**
Snack:		
½ cup fruit cup	70	**70**

Total Calories: 1,530

DAY 2 ▶ WEEK 2   Calories   Total Calories

Breakfast:

	Calories	Total Calories
*Open Face Melted Cheese Supreme (p. 194)	150	
*Frozen Orange Smiles (p. 200)	70	
½ cup low fat milk	60	**280**

Lunch:

	Calories	Total Calories
Pocket pita	80	
3 ounces turkey roll	150	
1 tbsp. light mayonnaise	40	
1 cup low fat milk	120	
Small green salad	50	
2 tbsp. low calorie dressing	25	**465**

Snack:

	Calories	Total Calories
1 apple, sliced	65	**65**

Dinner:

	Calories	Total Calories
*Thin Kids Fish Delight (p. 197)	315	
½ cup cooked rice	100	
½ cup mixed vegetables	60	
5 asparagus spears	15	
1 cup broth	50	
Small green salad	50	
2 tbsp. low calorie dressing	25	**615**

Snack:

	Calories	Total Calories
Low calorie ice cream pop	100	**100**

Total Calories: 1,525

DAY 3 ▶ WEEK 2

	Calories	Total Calories
Breakfast:		
½ cup cottage cheese	120	
*Thin Kids Fruited Milk Shake (p. 186)	200	**320**
Lunch:		
3 tbsp. peanut butter	315	
1 tbsp. low sugar jelly	15	
2 thin slices bread	80	
Raw vegetables	25	
*Frozen Banana Treat (p. 200)	80	**515**
Snack:		
1 cup low calorie yogurt	150	**150**
Dinner:		
4 ounces London broil	250	
1 medium potato, mashed	90	
1 tbsp. light margarine	50	
1 cup string beans	40	
Tossed salad	50	
2 tbsp. low calorie salad dressing	25	**505**
Snack:		
3 cups popcorn, popped	75	
1 tbsp. light margarine	50	**125**

Total Calories: 1,615

DAY 4 ▶ WEEK 2

	Calories	Total Calories
Breakfast:		
*Egg McPita (p. 183)	270	
½ grapefruit	45	
1 cup low fat milk	120	**435**
Lunch:		
*Thin Kids Pizza (p. 196)	320	
Sautéed vegetables	50	
1 pear	100	
1 cup low fat milk	120	**590**
Snack:		
*Thin Kids Ice Pop (p. 199)	100	**100**
Dinner:		
4 ounces chicken	200	
Small green salad	50	
2 tbsp. light salad dressing	25	
½ cup mixed vegetables	60	
Cucumber slices	30	
1 cup low calorie yogurt, whipped and frozen	150	
6 ounces tomato juice	35	**550**
Snack:		
½ cup strawberries	30	**30**
	Total Calories:	**1,705**

DAY 5 — WEEK 2

	Calories	Total Calories
Breakfast:		
1 rice cake	35	
1 tbsp. peanut butter	105	
1 cup low calorie yogurt	150	
1 orange	70	**360**
Lunch:		
3 ounces leftover chopped chicken added to tossed salad	200	
2 tbsp. low calorie dressing	25	
*Baked Apple Sweetness (p. 199)	85	
1 cup low fat milk	120	
1½ cup popped popcorn	40	**470**
Snack:		
6 ounces tomato juice	35	
Celery sticks	10	**45**
Dinner:		
4 ounces cooked shrimp	100	
4 ounces lamb patty	230	
½ cup wide noodles	100	
1 tbsp. light margarine	50	
3 broccoli spears	30	
Small green salad	50	
1 cup low fat milk	120	**680**
Snack:		
½ cup fruit cup	70	**70**

Total Calories: 1,625

DAY 6 — WEEK 2

	Calories	Total Calories
Breakfast:		
⅔ cup cereal	80	
1 cup low fat milk	120	
2 ounces riccota cheese	90	
½ cup strawberries	30	**320**
Lunch:		
Tuna salad sandwich:		
3 ounces tuna, chopped	165	
1 tbs. light mayonnaise	40	
3 tbsp. chopped celery	10	
1 pocket pita	80	
Lettuce and tomato	25	
1 apple	70	
1 cup low fat milk	120	**510**
Snack:		
½ cup peaches	50	**50**
Dinner:		
4 ounces roast beef	300	
1 medium potato, baked	90	
1 cup string beans	40	
1 tbsp. light margarine	50	
1 green salad	50	
2 tbsp. low calorie dressing	25	
½ cantaloupe	40	**595**
Snack:		
1 cup low calorie yogurt	150	**150**
	Total Calories:	**1,625**

DAY 7 — WEEK 2

	Calories	Total Calories
Breakfast:		
1 egg	80	
1 thin slice bread	40	
1 cup low fat milk	120	
1 orange	70	**310**
Lunch:		
*Toss The Log (p. 191)	350	
1 bread stick	35	
1 cup low fat milk	120	**505**
Snack:		
1 plum	75	**75**
Dinner:		
4 ounces cooked shrimp	100	
3 meat balls	300	
½ cup cooked pasta	100	
½ cup tomato sauce	50	
Fruit bowl:		
½ small banana	40	
¼ cup blueberries	25	
¼ cup strawberries	30	**645**
Snack:		
1½ cups popcorn, popped	40	
1 tbsp. light margarine	50	**90**

Total Calories: 1,625

WEEK THREE

DAY 1 ▶ WEEK 3   Calories   Total Calories

Breakfast:

	Calories	Total Calories
⅔ cup cereal	80	
½ cup low fat milk	60	
1 egg, scrambled	80	
1 tsp. light margarine	15	
½ grapefruit	45	**280**

Lunch:

	Calories	Total Calories
*Cold Tuna Pasta Salad (p. 191)	275	
Cucumber slices	10	
1 Tomato	25	
½ cup low fat milk	60	
1 peach	60	**430**

Snack:

	Calories	Total Calories
1 cup low calorie yogurt	150	**150**

Dinner:

	Calories	Total Calories
2 broiled lamb chops	240	
½ cup cooked rice	100	
½ cup carrots	25	
½ cup string beans	20	
Tossed salad	50	
2 tsp. light margarine	30	
2 tbsp. low calorie dressing	25	
6 ounces tomato or V-8 juice	35	
½ cup fruit cup	70	**595**

Snack:

	Calories	Total Calories
Low calorie ice cream pop	100	**100**

Total Calories: 1,555

DAY 2 ▶ WEEK 3

	Calories	Total Calories
Breakfast:		
½ thin bagel	100	
½ cup cottage cheese	120	
Tomato slices	25	
6 ounces orange juice	80	
1 cup low fat milk	120	**445**
Lunch:		
*Thin Kids Pizza (p. 196)	320	
½ cup sautéed vegetables	50	
1 4 ounce plum	75	**445**
Snack:		
1 cup chicken broth	50	
Raw vegetables and 2 tbsp. low calorie dressing	75	**125**
Dinner:		
4 ounces sliced turkey	200	
4 broccoli spears	40	
1 tbsp. light margarine	50	
Tossed salad	50	
2 tbsp. low calorie salad dressing	25	
*Thin Kids Fruited Milk Shake (p. 186)	200	**565**
Snack:		
1 cup low calorie yogurt	150	**150**
	Total Calories:	**1,730**

MENUS

DAY 3 ▶ WEEK 3

	Calories	Total Calories
Breakfast:		
*Open Face Melted Cheese Supreme (p. 194)	150	
1 cup low fat milk	120	
1 orange	70	**340**
Lunch:		
3 ounces sliced turkey	150	
2 thin slices bread	80	
1 tbsp. light mayonnaise	40	
1 pear	100	
Cucumber slices	15	
1 cup low calorie yogurt	150	**535**
Snack:		
Low calorie ice cream pop	100	**100**
Dinner:		
4 ounces roast beef	300	
1 medium potato, baked	90	
1 cup string beans	40	
Tossed salad	50	
1 tbsp. light margarine	50	
2 tbsp. low calorie salad dressing	25	
⅛ honeydew melon	55	**610**
Snack:		
1½ cups popcorn, popped	40	
1 cup tomato juice	35	**75**

Total Calories: 1,660

DAY 4 ▶ WEEK 3

	Calories	Total Calories
Breakfast:		
*Spinach Cheese Omelet Florentine (p. 184)	200	
1 cup low calorie yogurt	150	
1 orange	75	
1 slice thin bread	40	**465**
Lunch:		
*Cottage Cheese and Pear Platter (p. 192)	420	
3 crackers	45	
1 cup low fat milk	120	
1½ cups of popcorn, popped	40	**625**
Snack:		
1 low calorie ice cream pop	100	**100**
Dinner:		
*Orange Chicken Surprise (p. 197)	250	
½ cup carrots	25	
1 medium potato, baked	90	
Green salad	50	
1 tbsp. of light margarine	50	
2 tbsp. of low calorie dressing	25	
*Baked Apple Sweetness (p. 199)	85	**575**
Snack:		
*Frozen Banana Treat (p. 200)	80	**80**

Total Calories: 1,845

DAY 5 ▶ WEEK 3

	Calories	Total Calories
Breakfast:		
1 egg	80	
*Thin Kids Fruited Shake (p. 186)	200	
1 thin slice bread	40	**320**
Lunch:		
*Pink and Orange Salad (p. 192)	340	
Lettuce and Tomato	25	
Carrot sticks	25	
1 cup low fat milk	120	
1 peach	60	**570**
Snack:		
Chicken broth	50	
1½ cups popcorn, popped	40	**90**
Dinner:		
4 ounces veal burger	250	
½ cup spaghetti, cooked	100	
½ cup low calorie tomato sauce	50	
1 cup string beans	40	
Tossed salad	50	
2 tbsp. low calorie dressing	25	**515**
Snack:		
1 cup low calorie yogurt	150	**150**

Total Calories: 1,645

DAY 6 ▶ WEEK 3

	Calories	Total Calories
Breakfast:		
⅔ cup cereal	80	
1 slice cheese	110	
1 cup low fat milk	120	
½ cup strawberries	30	**340**
Lunch:		
1 cup cottage cheese	240	
½ cantaloupe	40	
½ cup sliced berries	35	
1 cup low fat milk	120	
2 crackers	35	
1 tsp. margarine	15	**485**
Snack:		
Low calorie ice cream pop	100	**100**
Dinner:		
*Chicken in the Pot (p. 196)	385	
1 cup green vegetables	40	
Salad	50	
2 tbsp. low calorie dressing	25	
1 cup tomato juice	35	**535**
Snack:		
*Thin Kids Ice Pops (p. 199)	90	**90**

Total Calories: 1,550

DAY 7 ▶ WEEK 3

	Calories	Total Calories
Breakfast:		
1 rice cake	35	
1 tbsp. peanut butter	105	
1 cup low calorie yogurt	150	
½ cup low fat milk	60	
*Frozen Orange Smiles (p. 200)	70	**420**
Lunch:		
1 cup chicken broth	50	
*Burger Build-Up (p. 193)	305	
½ cup fruit cup	70	**425**
Snack:		
1 cup low fat milk	120	**120**
Dinner:		
*Thin Kids Fish Delight (p. 197)	315	
1 cup vegetables	40	
1 medium potato, baked	90	
1 tbsp. light margarine	50	
1 small green salad	50	
2 tbsp. low calorie salad dressing	25	
1 cup vegetable juice	35	
*Baked Apple Sweetness (p. 199)	85	**690**
Snack:		
1½ cups popcorn, popped	40	
1 tbsp. light margarine	40	**80**

Total Calories: 1,735

WEEK FOUR

DAY 1 ▶ WEEK 4

	Calories	Total Calories
Breakfast:		
½ bagel	100	
½ cup cottage cheese	120	
Tomato slices	20	
½ grapefruit	45	
½ cup low fat milk	60	**345**
Lunch:		
1½ slices (ounces) roast beef roll-ups	120	
1½ slices (ounces) cheese roll-ups	150	
1 cup low calorie yogurt	150	
½ cup crushed pineapple	65	
Carrot and celery sticks	25	
1 cup low fat milk	120	**630**
Snack:		
1½ cups popcorn, popped	40	
1 cup tomato juice	35	**75**
Dinner:		
2 lamb chops, broiled	240	
½ cup cooked rice	100	
½ cup cooked carrots	25	
4 broccoli spears	40	
1 tbsp. light margarine	50	
Small green salad	50	
2 tbsp. low calorie dressing	25	**530**
Snack:		
*Thin Kids Ice Pop (p. 199)	90	**90**
	Total Calories:	**1,670**

DAY 2 ▶ WEEK 4

	Calories	Total Calories
Breakfast:		
1 thin slice bread	40	
1 tbsp. peanut butter	105	
1 cup low calorie yogurt	150	
6 ounces orange juice	80	**375**
Lunch:		
*Toss The Log Salad (p. 191)	350	
1 apple	70	
1 cup low fat milk	120	**540**
Snack:		
1 cup chicken broth	50	
2 crackers	35	**85**
Dinner:		
4 ounces cooked shrimp	100	
2 meat balls	200	
½ cup spinach	20	
1 medium potato, baked	90	
1 tbsp. light margarine	50	
Tomato and cucumber slices	35	
2 tbsp. low calorie dressing	25	
½ cantaloupe	40	
1 cup vegetable juice	35	**595**
Snack:		
Low calorie ice cream pop	100	**100**

Total Calories: 1,695

DAY 3 ▶ WEEK 4

	Calories	Total Calories

Breakfast:
1 egg	80	
1 tbsp. light margarine	40	
1 thin slice bread	50	
*Frozen Orange Smiles (p. 200)	70	
1 cup low fat milk	120	**360**

Lunch:
3 ounces leftover chicken	150	
Raw vegetables	25	
2 crackers	35	
¼ cantaloupe	20	
1 cup low fat milk	120	**350**

Snack:
*Frozen Grape Sensation (p. 200)	50	
1 cup chicken broth	50	**100**

Dinner:
4 ounces steak	260	
1 medium potato, baked	90	
1 cup string beans	40	
Green salad	50	
2 tbsp. low calorie dressing	25	
½ cup fruit cup	70	
1 cup low calorie yogurt	150	**685**

Snack:
1 cup tomato juice	35	
1½ cups popcorn, popped	40	**75**

Total Calories: 1,570

DAY 4 ▸ WEEK 4

	Calories	Total Calories
Breakfast:		
½ cup rice	100	
1 ounce cheese	110	
½ cantaloupe	40	
1 cup low fat milk	120	
1 tbsp. light margarine	50	**420**
Lunch:		
2 thin slices bread	80	
2 tbsp. peanut butter	210	
1 tbsp. low sugar jelly	15	
Carrot & celery sticks	25	
1 cup low fat milk	120	
1 nectarine	75	**525**
Snack:		
Low calorie ice cream pop	100	**100**
Dinner:		
*Thin Kids Fish Delight (p. 197)	315	
1 tbsp. light margarine	50	
½ cup mixed vegetables	60	
Green salad	50	
2 tbsp. low calorie dressing	25	
1 cup tomato juice	35	**535**
Snack:		
10 cherries	25	
10 grapes	25	**50**

Total Calories: 1,630

DAY 5 ▶ WEEK 4

	Calories	Total Calories
Breakfast:		
1 waffle	85	
1 tbsp. light margarine	50	
1 egg	80	
1 orange	70	
1 cup low fat milk	120	**405**
Lunch:		
Pocket pita	80	
3 ounces roast beef	240	
1 tbsp. light mayonnaise	40	
Lettuce and tomato	25	
Carrot and celery sticks	25	
1 cup vegetable juice	35	
1 cup low fat milk	120	**565**
Snack:		
*Thin Kids Ice Pop (p. 199)	90	**90**
Dinner:		
*Chicken in the Pot (p. 196)	385	
Green salad	50	
2 tbsp. low calorie dressing	25	
*Baked Apple Sweetness (p. 199)	85	**545**
Snack:		
1 cup low calorie yogurt	150	**150**
	Total Calories:	**1,755**

DAY 6 — WEEK 4

	Calories	Total Calories

Breakfast:
½ cup hot cereal	105	
1 small sliced banana	80	
1 cup low fat yogurt	150	
½ cup low fat milk	120	**455**

Lunch:
2 servings *Open Face Melted Cheese Supreme (p. 194)	300	
½ cup low fat milk	60	
Green salad	50	
2 tbsp low calorie dressing	25	**435**

Snack:
1 cup tomato juice	35	
1½ cups popcorn, popped	40	**75**

Dinner:
4 ounces cooked shrimp	100	
3 ounces filet of fish, broiled	180	
Green salad	50	
2 tsp. seafood sauce	25	
5 asparagus spears	15	
3 broccoli spears	30	
1 tbsp. light margarine	50	
2 tbsp. low calorie dressing	25	**475**

Snack:
Low calorie ice cream pop	100	**100**

Total Calories: 1,540

DAY 7 ▶ WEEK 4

	Calories	Total Calories
Breakfast:		
*Egg McPita (p. 183)	270	
½ grapefruit	45	
1 cup low fat milk	120	
1 tbsp. light margarine	50	**485**
Lunch:		
*Burger Build-Up (p. 193)	305	
Carrot and celery sticks	25	
1 cup tomato juice	35	
½ cantaloupe	40	**405**
Snack:		
1½ cups popcorn, popped	40	
*Thin Kids Ice Pop (p. 199)	120	**160**
Dinner:		
4 ounces roast turkey	200	
½ cup potato, mashed	100	
½ cup spinach	20	
½ cup cauliflower	15	
Green salad	50	
1 tbsp. light margarine	50	
2 tbsp. low calorie dressing	25	
1 cup low fat milk	120	**580**
Snack:		
1 cup sliced strawberries	60	**60**

Total Calories: 1,690

WEEK FIVE

DAY 1 — WEEK 5

	Calories	Total Calories
Breakfast:		
⅔ cup cereal	80	
1 cup low fat milk	120	
1 ounce cheese	105	
*Frozen Orange Smiles (p. 200)	70	**375**
Lunch:		
Tuna salad:		
½ cup tuna fish	165	
1 tbsp. light mayonnaise	40	
Chopped celery	15	
Lettuce and tomato	25	
Cucumber slices	15	
3 crackers	50	
1 cup vegetable juice	35	**345**
Snack:		
Low calorie ice cream pop	100	**100**
Dinner:		
4 ounces beef, broiled	250	
1 medium potato, baked	90	
Green salad	50	
1 cup broccoli	40	
1 cup low fat milk	120	
2 tbsp. low calorie salad dressing	50	
1 tbsp. light margarine	50	
½ cup fruit salad	70	**720**
Snack:		
½ grapefruit	45	**45**
Total Calories:		**1,585**

DAY 2 ▶ WEEK 5

	Calories	Total Calories
Breakfast:		
½ bagel	100	
1 egg	80	
½ tbsp. light margarine	25	
1 cup low fat milk	120	
½ grapefruit	45	**370**
Lunch:		
3 ounces turkey breast	150	
Pocket pita	80	
1 tbsp. light mayonnaise	40	
2 carrots	40	
Pear	100	
1 cup low fat milk	120	**530**
Snack:		
*Frozen Grape Sensation (p. 200)	50	
1 cup chicken broth	50	**100**
Dinner:		
*Thin Kids Fish Delight (p. 197)	315	
Green salad	50	
2 tbsp. low calorie dressing	25	
1 small potato, baked	50	
½ cup mixed vegetables	60	
1 cup low calorie yogurt	150	**650**
Snack:		
Green pepper and cucumber slices	25	**25**

Total Calories: 1,675

DAY 3 — WEEK 5

	Calories	Total Calories
Breakfast:		
½ cup hot cereal	105	
1 cup low fat milk	120	
½ cup cottage cheese	120	
*Frozen Banana Treat (p. 200)	80	**425**
Lunch:		
2 rice cakes	70	
2 tbsp. peanut butter	210	
Raw vegetables	25	
1 cup low fat milk	120	
1 apple	70	**495**
Snack:		
Low calorie ice cream pop	100	**100**
Dinner:		
½ cup spaghetti	100	
4 ounces chicken	200	
½ cup low calorie tomato sauce	50	
Salad	50	
2 tbsp. low calorie dressing	25	
1 cup strawberries	60	**485**
Snack:		
1 cup string beans	40	
1 tbsp. light margarine	50	**90**

Total Calories: 1,595

DAY 4 ▶ WEEK 5

	Calories	Total Calories
Breakfast:		
1 egg	80	
*Thin Kids Fruited Milk Shake (p. 186)	200	
1 thin slice bread	40	
1 tbsp. margarine	50	**370**
Lunch:		
*Reverse Sandwiches (p. 193)	350	
Carrot and celery sticks	25	
½ cantaloupe	40	
1 cup tomato juice	35	**450**
Snack:		
1 cup low calorie yogurt	150	**150**
Dinner:		
*Chicken in the Pot (p. 196)	385	
Green salad	50	
2 tbsp. low calorie dressing	25	
1 cup low fat milk	120	**585**
Snacks:		
½ cup fruit salad	70	**70**
	Total Calories:	**1,625**

DAY 5 ▶ WEEK 5

	Calories	Total Calories
Breakfast:		
½ small banana	40	
¼ ounce raisins	35	
½ cup cottage cheese	120	
1 cup low fat milk	120	
1 slice Melba toast	15	**330**
Lunch:		
1 thin slice bread	40	
½ cup canned salmon	165	
Chopped celery	15	
Lemon juice and vinegar for seasoning		
Lettuce and tomato	25	
1 peach	65	
1 cup low fat milk	120	**430**
Snack:		
Raw vegetables	25	
2 tbsp. low calorie dressing	25	
1 cup popcorn, popped	25	**75**
Dinner:		
4 ounces veal patty, broiled	245	
½ cup spaghetti	100	
½ cup low calorie tomato sauce	50	
Onions and green peppers, sautéed	50	
1 tbsp. light margarine	50	
Green salad	50	
2 tbsp. low calorie dressing	25	
½ cup fresh (or canned in water) pineapple	65	**635**
Snack:		
Low calorie ice cream pop	100	**100**

Total Calories: 1,570

DAY 6 — WEEK 5

	Calories	Total Calories
Breakfast:		
1 rice cake	35	
1 tbsp. peanut butter	105	
½ grapefruit	45	
1 cup low fat milk	120	**305**
Lunch:		
*Thin Kids Pizza (p. 196)	320	
1 cup low calorie yogurt	150	
½ cup strawberries	30	**500**
Snack:		
*Thin Kids Ice Pop (p. 199)	90	
1 cup chicken broth	50	**140**
Dinner:		
4 ounces shrimp, broiled	105	
3 ounces chicken	150	
½ cup rice	100	
1 cup string beans	40	
½ cup cooked carrots	25	
2 tbsp. light margarine	100	
Salad	50	
2 tbsp. low calorie dressing	25	
1 cup vegetable juice	35	**630**
Snack:		
*Frozen Grape Sensation (p. 200)	50	**50**

Total Calories: 1,625

DAY 7 — WEEK 5

	Calories	Total Calories
Breakfast:		
⅔ cup cereal	80	
1 cup low fat milk	120	
1 egg, scrambled	80	
1 tbsp. light margarine	50	
6 ounces orange juice	80	**410**
Lunch:		
2 thin slices bread	80	
3 ounces turkey breast	150	
1 tbsp. light mayonnaise	40	
1 tbsp. catsup	20	
Lettuce and tomato	25	
2 small plums	60	
1 cup low fat milk	120	**495**
Snack:		
1 cup low calorie yogurt	150	**150**
Dinner:		
4 ounces steak	260	
½ cup spinach	20	
½ cup peas and carrots	50	
Green salad	50	
2 tbsp. low calorie dressing	25	
1 cup tomato juice	35	
*Baked Apple Sweetness (p. 199)	85	**525**
Snack:		
1 cup chicken broth	50	
2 crackers	35	**85**

Total Calories: 1,665

WEEK SIX

DAY 1 — WEEK 6

	Calories	Total Calories
Breakfast:		
Bagelette	85	
1 tbsp. peanut butter	105	
1 tbsp. low sugar jelly	15	
1 cup low fat milk	120	
½ grapefruit	45	**370**
Lunch:		
Tossed salad with	50	
3 ounces turkey cubes	150	
2 tbsp. low calorie dressing	25	
1 bread stick	35	
1 cup low calorie yogurt	150	
½ cup crushed pineapple	65	**475**
Snack:		
2 cups popcorn, popped	50	
1 cup vegetable juice	35	**85**
Dinner:		
4 ounces roast beef	300	
1 medium potato, baked	90	
4 broccoli spears	40	
1 tbsp. light margarine	50	
Salad	50	
2 tbsp. low calorie dressing	25	
½ cup sliced peaches	50	**605**
Snack:		
Low calorie ice cream pop	100	**100**
	Total Calories:	**1,635**

MENUS

DAY 2 — WEEK 6

	Calories	Total Calories
Breakfast:		
1 thin slice bread	40	
*Thin Kids Fruited Milk Shake (p. 186)	200	
1 egg	80	**320**
Lunch:		
3 ounces chicken, chopped	150	
1 tbsp. light mayonnaise	40	
1 pocket pita	80	
Lettuce and tomato	25	
1 large carrot	25	
1 cup tomato juice	35	
¼ cantaloupe	20	**375**
Snack:		
1 cup low calorie yogurt	150	**150**
Dinner:		
1 cup chicken broth	50	
¼ cup rice	50	
2 lamp chops, broiled	240	
½ cup mixed vegetables	60	
1 medium potato, baked	90	
½ cup string beans	20	
Small green salad	25	
2 tbsp. low calorie dressing	25	
1 tbsp. light margarine	50	
1 cup strawberries	60	**670**
Snack:		
1 cup low fat milk	120	
10 black grapes	25	**145**

Total Calories: 1,660

DAY 3 ▶ WEEK 6

	Calories	Total Calories
Breakfast:		
⅔ cup cereal	80	
½ cup strawberries	30	
½ cup low fat milk	60	
*Frozen Orange Smiles (p. 200)	35	
½ cup cottage cheese	120	**325**
Lunch:		
3 ounces roast beef	240	
2 thin slices bread	80	
1 tbsp. light mayonnaise	40	
Lettuce and tomato	25	
Carrot and celery sticks	25	
1 peach	65	
1 cup low fat milk	120	**595**
Snack:		
Low calorie ice cream pop	100	**100**
Dinner:		
*Thin Kids Fish Delight (p. 197)	315	
1 medium potato, baked	90	
1 cup brussel sprouts	55	
½ cup cauliflower	15	
Green salad	50	
1 tbsp. light margarine	50	
2 tbsp. low calorie dressing	25	
1 cup tomato juice	35	**635**
Snack:		
1 cup melon balls	50	**50**

Total Calories: 1,705

DAY 4 — WEEK 6

	Calories	Total Calories

Breakfast:
*Open Face Melted Cheese Supreme (p. 194) — 150
1 cup low fat milk — 120
½ grapefruit — 45 — **315**

Lunch:
*Reverse Sandwiches (p. 193) — 350
1 cup low fat milk — 120
1 apple — 65 — **535**

Snack:
1 cup chicken broth — 50
2 crackers — 35 — **85**

Dinner:
4 ounces veal burger — 250
½ cup macaroni — 100
½ cup low calorie tomato sauce — 50
Sautéed mushrooms — 50
Salad — 50
2 tbsp. low calorie dressing — 25
20 cherries — 50 — **575**

Snack:
1 cup low calorie yogurt — 150 — **150**

Total Calories: 1,660

DAY 5 ▶ WEEK 6

	Calories	Total Calories
Breakfast:		
Poached egg	80	
Pocket pita	80	
1 orange	75	
1 cup low fat milk	120	**355**
Lunch:		
2 rice cakes	70	
2 tbsp. peanut butter	210	
1 cup low calorie yogurt	150	
1 apple	65	**495**
Snack:		
1½ cups popcorn, popped	40	
1 cup vegetable juice	35	**75**
Dinner:		
*Chicken in the Pot (p. 196)	385	
½ cucumber sliced with		
1 ounce sour cream	60	
1 cup string beans	40	
1 cup low fat milk	120	**605**
Snack:		
*Baked Apple Sweetness (p. 199)	85	**85**
	Total Calories:	**1,615**

DAY 6 ▸ WEEK 6

	Calories	Total Calories
Breakfast:		
1 thin slice bread	40	
2 ounces skim ricotta	90	
*Thin Kids Fruited Milk Shake (p. 186)	200	**330**
Lunch:		
*Thin Kids Pizza (p. 196)	320	
½ cup sautéed vegetables	50	
1 cup low fat milk	120	
Green salad	50	
2 tbsp. low calorie dressing	25	**565**
Snack:		
*Frozen Grape Sensation (p. 200)	50	**50**
Dinner:		
*Thin Kids Fish Delight (p. 197)	315	
1 medium potato, baked	90	
½ cup mixed vegetables	60	
4 broccoli spears	40	
Green salad	50	
2 tbsp. low calorie dressing	25	
1 tbsp. light margarine	50	
1 cup tomato juice	35	**665**
Snack:		
Low calorie ice cream pop	100	**100**
	Total Calories:	**1,705**

DAY 7 ▶ WEEK 6

	Calories	Total Calories
Breakfast:		
Soft boiled egg	80	
½ English muffin	75	
1 orange	75	
1 cup low fat milk	120	
½ tbsp. light margarine	25	**375**
Lunch:		
1 ounce cheese	110	
2 slices Melba toast	35	
*The Sticks (p. 200)	115	
Cherry tomatoes	25	
1 cup low fat milk	120	
½ cantaloupe	40	**445**
Snack:		
1 cup low calorie yogurt	150	**150**
Dinner:		
4 ounces turkey	200	
½ cup cabbage	15	
1 medium potato, baked	90	
Green salad	25	
1 tbsp. light margarine	50	
2 tbsp. low calorie dressing	25	
½ cup fruit salad	70	**475**
Snack:		
1½ cups popcorn, popped	40	
1 tbsp. light margarine	50	
1 cup vegetable juice	35	**125**

Total Calories: 1,570

WEEK SEVEN

DAY 1 ▸ WEEK 7	Calories	Total Calories
Breakfast:		
½ English muffin	75	
1 tbsp. peanut butter	105	
1 cup low calorie yogurt	150	
6 ounces orange juice	80	**410**
Lunch:		
4 ounces ricotta cheese	180	
Pocket pita	80	
1 apple	65	
Tomato and cucumber slices	25	
1 cup low fat milk	120	**470**
Snack:		
Low calorie ice cream pop	100	**100**
Dinner:		
4 ounces chicken breast	200	
1 artichoke, steamed	50	
1 cup broccoli	40	
1 medium potato, baked	90	
Salad	50	
2 tbsp. low calorie dressing	25	
1 tbsp. light margarine	50	
1 cup vegetable juice	35	**540**
Snack:		
½ cantaloupe	40	
3 sliced strawberries	15	**55**

Total Calories: 1,575

DAY 2 — WEEK 7

	Calories	Total Calories
Breakfast:		
⅔ cup cereal	80	
1 cup low fat milk	120	
*Hawaiian Whip (p. 183)	185	**385**
Lunch:		
Pocket pita	80	
3 ounces sliced turkey	150	
Lettuce and tomato	25	
2 tbsp. low calorie Russian dressing	25	
1 cup low fat milk	120	
1 peach	65	**465**
Snack:		
1 cup low calorie yogurt	150	**150**
Dinner:		
4 ounces lean pork chop with bone, broiled	230	
½ cup peas and carrots	45	
½ cup noodles	100	
1 cup string beans	40	
Salad	50	
2 tbsp. light margarine	100	
1 cup tomato juice	35	**600**
Snack:		
*Baked Apple Sweetness (p. 199)	85	**85**

Total Calories: 1,685

MENUS

DAY 3 ▶ WEEK 7

	Calories	Total Calories
Breakfast:		
Hard boiled egg	80	
1 tbsp. light mayonnaise	40	
Pocket pita	80	
½ grapefruit	45	
1 cup low fat milk	120	**365**
Lunch:		
*Toss The Log (p. 191)	350	
½ cup strawberries	30	
1 cup low fat milk	120	
2 tbsp. low calorie dressing	25	**525**
Snack:		
*Thin Kids Ice Pop (p. 199)	90	
1 cup chicken broth	50	**140**
Dinner:		
4 ounces veal burger	245	
½ cup eggplant	20	
½ cup string beans	20	
1 cup vegetable juice	35	
½ cup macaroni	100	
½ cup low calorie tomato sauce	50	**470**
Snack:		
1 cup low calorie yogurt	150	**150**
	Total Calories:	**1,650**

DAY 4 — WEEK 7

	Calories	Total Calories
Breakfast:		
1 cup low calorie yogurt	150	
1 tbsp. peanut butter	105	
1 rice cake	35	
½ cantaloupe	40	**330**
Lunch:		
*Meat Loaf Italiano sandwich (p. 195)	265	
Pocket Pita	80	
1 tbsp. catsup	20	
Lettuce and tomato	25	
1 large carrot	25	
2 tbsp. low calorie dressing	25	
1 cup low fat milk	120	**560**
Snack:		
2 small tangerines	80	**80**
Dinner:		
*Chicken in the Pot (p. 196)	385	
½ cup zucchini	15	
Green salad	50	
2 tbsp. low calorie dressing	25	
1 nectarine	75	**550**
Snack:		
Low calorie ice cream pop	100	**100**
	Total Calories:	**1,620**

DAY 5 — WEEK 7

	Calories	Total Calories

Breakfast:
2 ounces liver, broiled	75	
Carrots	25	
Celery	15	
1 pocket pita	80	
1 tbsp. cream cheese	30	
6 ounces orange juice	80	**305**

Lunch:
2 servings *Open Face Melted Cheese Supreme (p. 194)	300	
1 cup low calorie yogurt	150	
1 apple	65	**515**

Snack:
*Thin Kids Fruited Milk Shake (p. 186) (Strawberry)	200	**200**

Dinner:
4 ounces chicken	200	
1 cup zucchini and tomatoes	25	
¼ cup onions	15	
1 medium potato, baked	90	
Green salad	50	
1 tbsp. light margarine	50	
2 tbsp. low calorie dressing	25	**455**

Snack:
Low calorie ice cream pop	100	**100**

Total Calories: 1,575

DAY 6 — WEEK 7

	Calories	Total Calories
Breakfast:		
1 egg	80	
1 thin slice bread	40	
1 tbsp. light margarine	50	
1 cup low fat milk	120	
½ grapefruit	45	**335**
Lunch:		
Turkey and ham sandwich	280	
2 carrots	40	
6 ounces apple juice	100	**420**
Snack:		
1 cup low calorie yogurt	150	**150**
Dinner:		
3 meatballs	300	
½ cup low calorie tomato sauce	50	
½ cup spaghetti	100	
1 cup broccoli	40	
Green salad	50	
2 tbsp. low calorie dressing	25	
1 cup low fat milk	120	**685**
Snack:		
10 cherries	25	
*Frozen Grape Sensation (p. 200)	50	**75**

Total Calories: 1,665

DAY 7 ▶ WEEK 7

	Calories	Total Calories

Breakfast:
2 ounces ricotta cheese	90	
⅔ cup cereal	80	
½ cup low fat milk	60	
3 strawberries	15	**245**

Lunch:
3 ounces chicken breast	150	
Tossed salad	50	
2 tbsp. low calorie dressing	25	
1 cup low fat milk	120	
1 nectarine	75	**420**

Snack:
⅔ cup strawberries	45	
½ cup plain yogurt	75	**120**

Dinner:
*Thin Kids Pizza (p. 196)	320	
*Antipasto Salad (p. 190)	335	
Low calorie ice cream pop	100	**755**

Snack:
*Thin Kids Ice Pop (p. 199)	90	**90**

Total Calories: 1,630

WEEK EIGHT

DAY 1 — WEEK 8

	Calories	Total Calories
Breakfast:		
*Hawaiian Whip (p. 183)	185	
1 thin slice bread	40	
1 cup low fat milk	120	**345**
Lunch:		
*Peanuts and Pita (p. 193)	305	
1 orange	75	
1 cup low fat milk	120	
Carrot and celery sticks	25	**525**
Snack:		
1 cup chicken broth	50	
2 crackers	35	**85**
Dinner:		
*Thin Kids Fish Delight (p. 197)	315	
1 cucumber, sliced with		
1 tbsp. sour cream	60	
1 cup string beans	40	
Corn on the cob, 3 inch ear	85	
Green salad	50	
2 tbsp. low calorie dressing	25	
1 tbsp. light margarine	50	**625**
Snack:		
1 cup melon balls	50	
1 cup low calorie yogurt	150	**200**

Total Calories: 1,780

DAY 2 ▶ WEEK 8

	Calories	Total Calories

Breakfast:
1 egg, scrambled	80	
½ tbsp. light margarine	25	
1 cup low calorie yogurt	150	
½ grapefruit	45	**300**

Lunch:
*Burger Build-Up (p. 193) (3 ounce hamburger)	305	
1 cup low fat milk	120	
1 peach	65	**490**

Snack:
1½ cups popcorn, popped	40	
½ tbsp. light margarine	25	
1 cup vegetable juice	35	**100**

Dinner:
4 ounces turkey	200	
Sautéed mushrooms	50	
½ cup broccoli and carrots, mixed	45	
½ cup potatoes, mashed	100	
Green salad	50	
1 tbsp. light margarine	50	
2 tbsp. low calorie dressing	25	
*Frozen Grape Sensation (p. 200)	50	**570**

Snack:
*Low calorie ice cream pop	100	**100**

Total Calories: 1,560

DAY 3 ▶ WEEK 8

	Calories	Total Calories
Breakfast:		
*Open Face Melted Cheese Supreme (p. 194)	150	
6 ounces apple juice	100	**250**
Lunch:		
3 ounces turkey	150	
1 cup chicken broth	50	
Tossed salad	50	
2 tbsp. low calorie dressing	25	
1 cup low fat milk	120	
1 peach	65	**460**
Snack:		
1 cup low calorie yogurt	150	**150**
Dinner:		
4 ounces veal chop, broiled	265	
Sautéed onions and peppers	50	
1 tbsp. light margarine	50	
½ cup noodles	100	
½ cup low calorie tomato sauce	50	
Salad	50	
2 tbsp. low calorie dressing	25	
2 small tangerines	80	**670**
Snack:		
1 cup low fat milk	120	
3 cups popcorn, popped	75	**195**

Total Calories: 1,725

DAY 4 ▶ WEEK 8

	Calories	Total Calories
Breakfast:		
1 rice cake	35	
1 tbsp. peanut butter	105	
1 cup low calorie yogurt	150	
*Frozen Orange Smiles (p. 200)	75	
½ cup low fat milk	60	**425**
Lunch:		
Roast Beef Sandwich:		
3 ounces roast beef	240	
1 pocket pita	80	
Lettuce and tomato	25	
2 tbsp. low calorie dressing	25	
Raw vegetables	25	
1 cup low fat milk	120	
1 apple	65	**580**
Snack:		
*2 Thin Kids Pops (p. 199)	200	**200**
Dinner:		
*Thin Kids Fish Delight (p. 197)	315	
½ cup rice	100	
5 asparagus spears	15	
½ cup carrots, cooked	25	
Salad	50	
2 tbsp. low calorie dressing	25	
½ cup low fat milk	60	**590**
Snack:		
1 cup chicken broth	50	
1 bread stick	35	**85**

Total Calories: 1,880

DAY 5 ▶ WEEK 8

	Calories	Total Calories
Breakfast:		
½ English muffin	75	
2 ounces ricotta cheese	90	
Tomato slices	15	
1 cup low fat milk	120	
½ cantaloupe	40	**340**
Lunch:		
*Pink and Orange Salad (p. 192)	325	
1 cup vegetable juice	35	
½ cup strawberries	30	**390**
Snack:		
Low calorie ice cream pop	100	**100**
Dinner:		
4 ounces roast beef	300	
½ cup spinach	25	
½ cup string beans	20	
1 medium potato, baked	90	
1 tbsp. light margarine	50	
Salad	50	
2 tbsp. low calorie dressing	25	
*Frozen Grape Sensation (p. 200)	25	**585**
Snack:		
1 cup low fat milk	120	
*Frozen Banana Treat (p. 200)	80	**200**

Total Calories: 1,615

DAY 6 — WEEK 8

	Calories	Total Calories
Breakfast:		
1 egg	80	
1 mini bagel	85	
1 tbsp. light margarine	50	
1 orange	75	
1 cup low fat milk	120	**410**
Lunch:		
½ cup pasta	100	
2 meatballs	200	
½ cup tomato sauce	50	
½ cucumber, sliced	15	
Plum	75	**440**
Snack:		
1 cup low calorie yogurt	150	**150**
Dinner:		
*Thin Kids Fish Delight (p. 197)	315	
4 broccoli spears	40	
½ cup carrots, cooked	25	
1 cup Brussels sprouts	40	
½ cup rice	100	
1 tbsp. light margarine	50	
1 cup low fat milk	120	**690**
Snack:		
½ cup fruit cup	70	**70**

Total Calories: 1,760

DAY 7 ▸ WEEK 8

	Calories	Total Calories
Breakfast:		
⅔ cup cereal	80	
½ cup low fat milk	60	
½ cup strawberries	30	
½ cup cottage cheese	120	**290**
Lunch:		
*Reverse Sandwiches (p. 193)	350	
1 cup low fat milk	120	
½ cup applesauce	50	**520**
Snack:		
Low calorie ice cream pop	100	**100**
Dinner:		
*Chicken Parmesan (p. 196)	350	
½ cup spaghetti	100	
½ cup low calorie tomato sauce	50	
Salad	50	
1 cup broccoli	40	
2 tbsp. low calorie dressing	25	
1 tbsp. light margarine	50	**665**
Snack:		
1½ cups popcorn, popped	40	
1 cup tomato juice	35	**75**

Total Calories: 1,650

WEEK 9

DAY 1 — WEEK NINE

	Calories	Total Calories
Breakfast:		
1 pancake	95	
1 egg	80	
1 tbsp. light margarine	50	
1 orange	75	
1 cup low fat milk	120	**420**
Lunch:		
2 thin slices bread	80	
2 tbsp. peanut butter	210	
1 tbsp. low sugar jelly	15	
Carrot and celery sticks	25	
1 cup low fat milk	120	
1 apple	65	**515**
Snack:		
1 cup chicken broth	50	**50**
Dinner:		
4 ounces veal meatballs	320	
½ cup cooked macaroni	100	
½ cup low calorie tomato sauce	50	
½ cup squash	35	
Green salad	50	
2 tbsp. low calorie dressing	25	**580**
Snack:		
1 cup low calorie yogurt	150	
½ cup fruit cup	70	**220**

Total Calories: 1,785

DAY 2 ▶ WEEK 9

	Calories	Total Calories
Breakfast:		
1 rice cake	35	
1 ounce cheese	110	
1 cup low calorie yogurt	150	
6 ounces orange juice	80	**375**
Lunch:		
3 ounces chopped chicken	150	
2 thin slices bread	80	
1 tbsp. light mayonnaise	40	
Lettuce and tomato	25	
Pepper slices	15	
1 cup low fat milk	120	
½ cup strawberries	30	
1 cup popcorn, popped	25	**485**
Snack:		
*Frozen Grape Sensation (p. 200)	50	**50**
Dinner:		
4 ounces minute steak	240	
1 tomato, 1 onion, and ½ cucumber	40	
½ cup carrots	25	
5 asparagus spears	15	
1 medium potato, baked	90	
Salad	50	
1 tbsp. light margarine	50	
2 tbsp. low calorie dressing	25	
1 low calorie ice cream	100	**635**
Snack:		
½ cup strawberries with 1 tbsp. sour cream	60	
1 small banana, sliced	80	**140**

Total Calories: 1,685

DAY 3 — WEEK 9

	Calories	Total Calories
Breakfast:		
1¼ ounce waffle	85	
1 tbsp. light margarine	50	
½ cup cottage cheese	120	
*Frozen Banana Treat (p. 200)	80	
1 cup low fat milk	120	**455**
Lunch:		
3 ounces cooked turkey	150	
1 pocket pita	80	
Lettuce and tomato	25	
1 tbsp. light mayonnaise	40	
1 orange	75	
1 cup popcorn, popped	25	
1 cup low fat milk	120	**515**
Snack:		
1 cup low calorie yogurt	150	**150**
Dinner:		
*Chicken in the Pot (p. 196)	385	
½ portion green salad	25	
2 tbsp. low calorie dressing	25	
1 apple	65	**500**
Snack:		
1 cup tomato juice	35	
Raw vegetables	25	**60**

Total Calories: 1,680

DAY 4 — WEEK 9

	Calories	Total Calories
Breakfast:		
½ cup hot cereal	105	
½ small banana, sliced	40	
1 cup low fat milk	120	
1 egg	80	**345**
Lunch:		
3 ounces roast beef	240	
2 thin slices bread	80	
Lettuce and tomato	25	
1 tbsp. light mayonnaise	40	
1 cup low calorie yogurt	150	
1 cup low fat milk	120	
1 apple	65	**720**
Snack:		
2 small tangerines	80	**80**
Dinner:		
4 ounces veal chops, broiled	265	
½ cup rice	100	
½ cup squash	35	
½ cup broccoli	20	
Salad	50	
1 tbsp. light margarine	50	
2 tbsp. low calorie dressing	25	**540**
Snack:		
1 4 inch by 6 inch watermelon wedge	90	**90**
	Total Calories:	**1,775**

DAY 5 — WEEK 9

	Calories	Total Calories
Breakfast:		
1 rice cake	35	
1 tbsp. cream cheese	30	
1 ounce cheese	110	
1 cup low calorie yogurt	150	
1 orange	75	**400**
Lunch:		
*Reverse Sandwiches (p. 193)	350	
1 cup low fat milk	120	
1 peach	65	**535**
Snack:		
½ cantaloupe	40	**40**
Dinner:		
2 lamb chops, broiled	240	
1 medium potato, baked	90	
5 asparagus spears	15	
½ cup cauliflower	15	
Green salad	50	
1 cup tomato juice	35	
Low calorie ice cream pop	100	
2 tbsp. low calorie dressing	25	**570**
Snack:		
3 cups popcorn, popped	75	**75**

Total Calories: 1,620

DAY 6 ▶ WEEK 9

	Calories	Total Calories
Breakfast:		
1 thin slice bread	40	
1 tbsp. peanut butter	105	
*Thin Kids Fruited Milk Shake, with banana (p. 186)	200	**345**
Lunch:		
*Sea and Roost Salad in Pita (p. 194)	300	
½ cantaloupe	40	
1 cup low fat milk	120	
½ cucumber, sliced	15	**475**
Snack:		
1 cup low calorie yogurt	150	**150**
Dinner:		
1 cup chicken broth	50	
4 ounces Cornish hen	200	
½ cup noodles	100	
½ cup brussel sprouts	25	
½ cup carrots	25	
Green salad	50	
1 tbsp. light margarine	50	
2 tbsp. low calorie dressing	25	
1 cup vegetable juice	35	**560**
Snack:		
½ grapefruit	45	**45**

Total Calories: 1,575

DAY 7 — WEEK 9

	Calories	Total Calories
Breakfast:		
1 egg	80	
1 mini bagel	85	
1 tbsp. light margarine	50	
1 cup low fat milk	120	
½ grapefruit	45	**380**
Lunch:		
*Thin Kids Pizza (p. 196)	320	
½ cup sautéed vegetables	50	
1 cup low fat milk	120	
1 cup honeydew melon	55	**545**
Snack:		
1 cup low calorie yogurt	150	**150**
Dinner:		
4 ounces scallops, broiled	125	
1 medium potato, boiled	90	
Cucumber slices	15	
Lettuce and tomato	25	
1 cup string beans	40	
½ cup zucchini	30	
1 cup tomato juice	35	
1 tbsp. light margarine	50	**410**
Snack:		
Tossed salad	50	
2 tbsp. low calorie dressing	25	**75**

Total Calories: 1,560

WEEK TEN

DAY 1 — WEEK 10

	Calories	Total Calories
Breakfast		
⅔ cup cereal	80	
1 cup low fat milk	120	
1 ounce cheese	110	
1 orange	75	**385**
Lunch:		
1 cup cottage cheese	240	
½ cantaloupe	40	
3 sliced strawberries	15	
3 crackers	45	
1 cup low fat milk	120	
Carrot and celery sticks	25	**485**
Snack:		
1 cup chicken broth	50	
2 crackers	35	**85**
Dinner:		
4 ounces veal cutlet	250	
4 broccoli spears	40	
½ cup carrots	25	
1 medium potato, baked	90	
Salad	50	
1 tbsp. light margarine	50	
2 tbsp. low calorie dressing	25	
½ cup fruit cup	70	**600**
Snack:		
1 low calorie ice cream pop	100	**100**

Total Calories: 1,655

DAY 2 — WEEK 10

	Calories	Total Calories
Breakfast:		
1 egg	80	
*Thin Kids Fruited Milk Shake (p. 186)	200	
1 thin slice bread	40	**320**
Lunch:		
*Chicken in the Pot (p. 196)	385	
1 pear	100	
1 cup low fat milk	120	**605**
Snack:		
1½ cups popcorn, popped	40	
1 tbsp. light margarine	50	**90**
Dinner:		
*Meat Loaf Italiano (p. 195)	265	
½ cup spaghetti	100	
½ cup low calorie tomato sauce	50	
1 cup cauliflower	30	
1 tbsp. light margarine	50	
Green salad	50	
2 tbsp. low calorie dressing	25	**570**
Snack:		
1 cup low fat yogurt	150	**150**

Total Calories: 1,735

DAY 3 ▶ WEEK 10

	Calories	Total Calories
Breakfast:		
*Hawaiian Whip with ½ cup cottage cheese (p. 183)	185	
2 rice cakes	70	
1 cup low fat milk	120	**375**
Lunch:		
4 ounces ricotta cheese	180	
Pocket pita	80	
Raw vegetables	25	
2 tbsp. low calorie dressing	25	
1 apple	65	
1 cup low fat milk	120	**495**
Snack:		
6 ounces *Orange Slush (p. 186)	80	**80**
Dinner:		
4 ounces steak	240	
½ cup carrots	25	
½ cup string beans	20	
½ cup cooked rice	100	
1½ tbsp. light margarine	75	
Green salad	50	
2 tbsp. low calorie dressing	25	
1 cup vegetable juice	35	**570**
Snack:		
1 cup low calorie yogurt	150	**150**

Total Calories: 1,670

DAY 4 ▸ WEEK 10

	Calories	Total Calories
Breakfast:		
½ cup hot oatmeal	105	
¼ cup raisins	65	
Cinnamon		
1 cracker	15	
1 tbsp. peanut butter	105	**290**
Lunch:		
*Pink and Orange Salad (p. 192)	325	
1 cup low fat milk	120	
1 peach	65	**510**
Snack:		
1 cup low calorie yogurt	150	**150**
Dinner:		
1 cup chicken broth	50	
4 ounces chicken	200	
1 medium potato, baked	90	
5 asparagus spears	15	
½ cup mixed vegetables	60	
Green salad	50	
2 tbsp. low calorie dressing	25	
1 cup tomato juice	35	
Low calorie ice cream pop	100	**625**
Snack:		
*Frozen Grape Sensation (p. 200)	50	**50**

Total Calories: 1,625

DAY 5 — WEEK 10

	Calories	Total Calories
Breakfast:		
*Open Face Melted Cheese Supreme (p. 194)	150	
*Frozen Orange Smiles (p. 200)	75	
½ cup low fat milk	60	**285**
Lunch:		
Pocket pita	80	
3 ounces turkey roll	150	
Green salad	50	
2 tbsp. low calorie dressing	25	
1 cup low fat milk	120	**425**
Snack:		
½ cantaloupe	40	**40**
Dinner:		
*Thin Kids Fish Delight (p. 197)	315	
1 medium potato, baked	90	
5 asparagus spears	15	
½ cup mixed vegetables	60	
1 cup chicken broth	50	
*Baked Apple Sweetness (p. 199)	85	
Green salad	50	
2 tbsp. low calorie dressing	25	
1 tbsp. light margarine	50	**740**
Snack:		
Low calorie ice cream pop	100	**100**
	Total Calories:	**1,590**

MENUS

DAY 6 ▶ WEEK 10

	Calories	Total Calories
Breakfast		
⅔ cup cereal	80	
1 cup low fat milk	120	
1 egg	80	
1 tbsp. light margarine	50	**330**
Lunch:		
3 ounces sliced chicken	150	
2 thin slices bread	80	
Lettuce and tomato	25	
Raw vegetables	25	
1 apple	65	
1 cup low fat milk	120	**465**
Snack:		
6 ounces *Orange Slush (p. 200)	80	**80**
Dinner:		
1 serving *Meat Loaf Italiano (p. 195)	320	
1 medium potato, baked	90	
½ cup cauliflower	15	
½ cup broccoli	15	
Green salad	50	
1 tbsp. light margarine	50	
2 tbsp. low calorie dressing	25	
1 cup low calorie yogurt	150	
1 cup vegetable juice	35	**695**
Snack:		
*1 Thin Kids Ice Pops (p. 199)	90	**90**
	Total Calories:	**1,660**

DAY 7 ▶ WEEK 10 — Calories / Total Calories

Breakfast:
½ English muffin	75	
1 tbsp. peanut butter	105	
1 cup low fat milk	120	
½ cup peaches	50	**350**

Lunch:
*Toss The Log Salad (p. 191)	350	
1 cup low fat milk	120	
1 apple	65	**535**

Snack:
Low calorie ice cream pop	100	**100**

Dinner:
4 ounces veal burger	250	
½ cup pasta, cooked	100	
1 low calorie tomato sauce	50	
½ cup sautéed onions and peppers	50	
1 cup string beans	40	
Green salad	50	
1 tbsp. light margarine	50	
2 tbsp. low calorie dressing	25	
½ cup fruit cup	70	**685**

Snack:
3 cups popcorn, popped	75	
1 cup tomato juice	35	**110**

Total Calories: 1,780

CHAPTER XIII

Thin Kids Recipe Section

This chapter contains all you need to know plus more about making the special Thin Kids dishes starred in the preceding menus. Just look up the dish you need, follow the instructions exactly regarding weights and measurements of ingredients, and enjoy a delicious low calorie meal designed just for you.

Breakfasts and Brunches **183**

Beverages **186**

Soups **188**

Salads **190**

Sandwiches **193**

Main Dishes **195**

Dressings and Sauce **198**

Desserts **199**

Snacks **200**

RECIPES

BREAKFASTS AND BRUNCHES

COTTAGE CHEESE MORNING DANISH

	Calories
½ English muffin	75
½ cup cottage cheese	120
¼ oz. raisins	40
Sprinkle of cinnamon	

Combine cottage cheese, raisins and sprinkle of cinnamon. Spoon onto ½ English muffin and bake for 15 minutes at 350 degrees.

Serves one   Total calories: **235**

THE HAWAIIAN WHIP

	Calories
1 cup cottage cheese	240
½ cup crushed pineapple	60
2 tbsp. pineapple juice	10

In blender, add cottage cheese, crushed pineapple, and pineapple juice. Blend until creamy.

Serves one   Calories per serving: **310**

EGG McPITA

	Calories
1 pocket pita	80
1 egg	80
1 ounce cheese	110

Soft boil or fry egg sunny side up in Silverstone skillet. Place in pocket pita along with favorite cheese. (Optional: Bake at 350 degrees for 10 minutes.)

Serves one   Total calories: **270**

POPULAR PANCAKES

	Calories
¼ cup all-purpose flour	100
½ cup non-fat dry milk	40
2 eggs	160
⅛ tsp. salt	
Dash of nutmeg	
Dash of cinnamon	

Mix flour with dry milk until smooth and without lumps. Beat eggs into milk. Stir in spices. Cook in Silverstone skillet sprayed with non-stick spray until brown on both sides; repeat with other side.

Serves three   Calories per serving: **95**

SPINACH CHEESE OMELET FLORENTINE

	Calories
1 egg	80
1 tbsp. water	
½ ounce shredded cheese	65
¼ cup spinach	5
1 tbsp. light margarine (optional)*	50

Chop, cook and drain spinach. Lightly beat egg with water. Spray small Silverstone skillet with non-stick cooking spray and melt margarine. Add egg and cook slowly. When egg is almost set, add cheese and spinach. Fold over omelet.

Serves one   Calories per serving: **200**

*for added flavor

LASAGNA STYLE OMELET

	Calories
1 egg	80
1 tbsp. water	
¼ cup cottage cheese or ¼ cup ricotta cheese	60
1 tbsp. Parmesan cheese	20
Dash of oregano	25
¼ cup low calorie tomato sauce	25
1 tbsp. light margarine (optional)*	50

Lightly beat egg with water. Spray small Silverstone skillet with non-stick cooking spray and melt margarine. Add egg. When egg begins to set, spread cottage cheese or ricotta cheese and 1 tsp. of the Parmesan cheese over egg and sprinkle on oregano. Fold over omelet and cook until cheese mixture is hot. Remove omelet from skillet and pour heated tomato sauce on top. Sprinkle with remaining Parmesan cheese.

Serves one   Calories per serving: **260**

*for added flavor

BEVERAGES

SUNSHINE MORNING DRINK

	Calories
3 cups orange juice	270
1 egg	80
2 tbsp. honey	120
Dash of nutmeg	

Combine ingredients in blender and whip for 30 seconds, or mix with rotary beater.
Serves four   Calories per serving: **117**

THIN KIDS FRUITED MILK SHAKE

	Calories
1 cup low fat milk	120
1 cup strawberries or 1 small banana	80
3 ice cubes	
½ tsp. vanilla	

Combine milk, fruit, ice and vanilla in a blender. Blend well for one minute.
Serves one   Total calories: **200**

ORANGE SLUSH*

	Calories
6 ounces orange juice	80

Pour orange juice into paper cup. Freeze for 45 minutes to 1 hour. Remove from freezer. (Optional: Blend for 10 seconds.)
Serves one   Total calories: **80**

*Other unsweetened juices may also be used.

RECIPES

GRAPE SPRITZER

	Calories
6 ounces grape juice*	120
4 ounces seltzer	

Pour grape juice into tall glass. Pour in seltzer and ice. Stir and enjoy.

Serves one Calories per serving: **120**

*Orange juice may also be used.

CRANBERRY COOLER FOR PARTIES

	Calories
46 ounce can of unsweetened cranberry-apple juice	850
2 tbsp. of lemon juice	15
6 ounce can of frozen orange juice concentrate	360
10 ounce bottle of seltzer, chilled	

Mix juice and frozen orange juice concentrate. Chill. Add chilled seltzer just before serving. A 6 ounce serving equals one fruit serving.

Serves twelve Calories per serving: Approximately **102**

SOUPS

COLD ANYTIME GAZPACHO

	Calories
2 small onions, finely chopped	20
1 garlic clove, crushed	
5 tomatoes, peeled and chopped	150
2 medium green peppers, chopped	25
2 cucumbers, chopped	60
1 cup chicken broth	50
3 tablespoons red vinegar	10
1/4 tsp. black pepper	

Mix onion, garlic and all but one cup of the tomatoes in blender until smooth. Then blend in half of the green pepper, half of the cucumber, broth, oil, vinegar and pepper until smooth. Chill for at least one hour. When serving, combine the remaining cucumbers, peppers, onions, and tomatoes. Divide into six portions. Pour blended mixture on top and serve as a cold soup anytime.

Serves 6   Calories per serving: **50**

*ANYTIME CHICKEN SOUP   Calories

1½ qts. water
2½ lbs. chicken, quartered
1 package soup greens
1 packet chicken bouillon powder

Bring water to boil. Add remaining ingredients. Bring to second boil. Reduce heat and simmer for 1½ hours. Pour off chicken broth. Store remaining chicken and vegetables in refrigerator. Refrigerate soup and skim off fat. Then re-heat and serve.

Yield: Two quarts   Calories per serving: **50**

*This soup is also an ingredient for Chicken-in-the-Pot, and can be used as a snack.

ANYTIME VEGETABLE SOUP   Calories
Method I—Using fresh vegetables
    2 potatoes, peeled and sliced   150
    ½ cup green beans, chopped   25
    ½ cup onion, chopped   20
    Any other fresh vegetables desired
    Seasoning to taste
    1 46 ounce can of vegetable juice   270
    5¾ cup water

Method II—Using frozen vegetables
    1 10 ounce package mixed frozen vegetables

Pour juice (see Method I) into a large pot. Fill empty can with water and add to juice. Bring to boil. Add vegetables and bring to a second boil. Simmer for 20 minutes or until vegetables soften. Terrific anytime!

Yield: 14–15 cups   Calories per serving: **40**

SALADS

ANTIPASTO SALAD

	Calories
1 cup lettuce, shredded	25
½ tomato, sliced	10
¼ pepper, cut in strips	10
¼ cucumber, sliced	10
2 mushrooms, sliced	10
1 ounce provolone cheese, sliced or diced	90
1 ounce ham, sliced or diced	50
1 ounce Italian salami, sliced or diced	115
2 tbsp. low calorie Italian dressing	25

Combine salad ingredients. Top with cheese, ham and salami. Toss with Italian salad dressing.

Serves one   Total calories: **335**

TOMATOES ALL DRESSED UP

	Calories
6 tomatoes	180
½ cup cooked white rice	100
1 tbsp. minced onion	10
1 cup small frozen peas, cooked and drained	100
⅛ tsp. salt	
¼ tsp. of pepper	

Cut off tomato tops ¼ inches from top. Using a teaspoon, scoop out inside of tomato, reserving pulp. Sprinkle a dash of salt in each of the hollowed tomatoes. Turn upside down and let stand. Meanwhile, mix together the rice, minced onions, peas and tomato pulp with the pepper. Spoon rice mixture into each tomato. Serve slightly chilled.

Serves 6   Calories per serving: **65**

COLD TUNA PASTA SALAD

                                                                  Calories

Ingredient	Calories
½ cup cold pasta	100
½ cup tuna drained and flaked	165
2 teaspoons low calorie Italian dressing	10
Dash of oregano	

Combine all ingredients in a medium-size bowl. Chill in refrigerator, covered, for a couple of hours before serving.

Serves one   Total calories: **275**

STUFFED TOMATO SURPRISE

Ingredient	Calories
3 ounces chopped chicken	150
1 tbsp. light mayonnaise	40
1 large ripe tomato	50
2 crackers	35
Optional: Celery, if desired	

Remove center core from ripe tomato. Add 4 more slits to top of tomato. Stuff chicken salad into tomato center. Serve with 2 crackers.

Serves one   Total calories: **275**

TOSS THE LOG

1½ cup favorite salad ingredients:

Ingredient	Calories
1 ounce turkey	50
1 ounce roast beef	75
1 ounce ham	50
1 ounce cheese	100
2 tbsp. favorite low calorie dressing	25

Layer meats and cheese, then roll into log. Slice log into ½ inch sections and place on salad, adding 2 tbsp. of your favorite low calorie dressing.

Serves one   Total calories: **300**

CUCUMBERS ALL DRESSED UP

                                               Calories

6 tsp. of salad oil	175
1 tbsp. white vinegar	
1 tsp. dry dill weed	
⅛ tsp. pepper	
1 cucumber, chopped	30
Optional: 2 thin onion slices	20

Combine first four ingredients. Slice cucumber thinly and cover with small onion slices, if desired. Cover with Oo-La-La Frenchette dressing (see p. 198) and chill for 3 hours.

Serves one   Calories per serving: **225**

PINK AND ORANGE SALAD
(Tuna and Carrot Salad)

                                                 Calories

3 ounces chopped, water-packed tuna	165
1 carrot, shredded	25
1 tbsp. light mayonnaise	40
2 slices of thin rye bread	80

Mix first three ingredients in large bowl. Spread on one slice of bread. Add lettuce and tomato, if desired.

Serves one   Calories per serving: **310**

COTTAGE CHEESE AND PEAR PLATTER

                                                 Calories

1 cup cottage cheese	240
⅛ cup raisins	60
1 tbsp. light mayonnaise	40
Dash of cinnamon	
½ cup pear halves	60
2 lettuce leaves	10

Combine first 3 ingredients with cinnamon. Place pear halves on lettuce beds. Scoop cottage cheese mixture into pear centers.

Serves one   Calories per serving: **410**

RECIPES

SANDWICHES

BURGER BUILD-UP

	Calories
1 hamburger bun	100
3 to 4 oz. cooked hamburger meat	250
2 lettuce leaves	5
2 tomato slices	10
4 pickle chips	10
1 tbsp. catsup	20
1 tsp. mustard	5

Remove some breading from inner bun. Mix mustard and catsup together. Place hamburger on bottom of bun. Add catsup mixture. Layer pickles, tomato, and lettuce. Cover with top of bun.
Special note: 3 oz. burger = 305 calories (lunch)
              4 oz. burger = 400 calories (dinner)
Serves one

REVERSE SANDWICHES

	Calories
3 breadsticks	100
3 ounces favorite protein, such as cheese, roast beef, chicken, etc.	250

Wrap slices of favorite protein around breadstick. Optional: Add mayonnaise or mustard between meat and breadstick.
Serves one   Calories per serving: **350**

PEANUTS AND PITAS

	Calories
2 tbsp. peanut butter	210
1 tsp. low sugar jelly	15
1 pita bread	80

Spoon peanut butter and low sugar jelly into pocket pita. Serve.
                              Calories per serving: **305**

SEA AND ROOST SALAD IN PITA

	Calories
1 pocket pita	80
1½ ounces of tuna, water-packed	85
1 tbsp. light mayonnaise	40
1 hard boiled egg	80
2 tablespoons of celery (optional)	
Lettuce, tomato, alfalfa sprouts	5

Mix all ingredients in a bowl. Stuff salad into pita with chopped lettuce, tomato, and alfalfa sprouts, if desired.
Serves one   Calories per serving: **290**

OPEN FACE MELTED CHEESE SUPREME

	Calories
1 thin slice bread	40
1 ounce cheese	100
2 tomato slices (optional)	10

Place 1 oz. of your favorite cheese on 1 slice of thin bread toast, placing tomato (if desired) between cheese and bread. Bake for 15 minutes or until cheese is well melted.

Serves one
Total calories: **150**

THIN AND CHEESY

	Calories
2 ounces of your favorite cheese slices	210
Mustard or light mayonnaise	40
Lettuce and tomato	20
2 thin slices bread	80

Mix favorite cheese slices with mustard or mayonnaise. Place on thin bread with lettuce and tomato.
Serves one   Calories per serving: **300–350**

RECIPES

MAIN DISHES

MEAT LOAF ITALIANO

	Calories
1 cup salt-free canned tomatoes	45
1 lb. lean ground beef	800
1 onion	20
2 dashes of garlic powder	
t tsp. oregano	
1 egg	80
¼ cup bread crumbs (optional)	115

Drain tomatoes and save tomato juice. Finely chop tomatoes and onion. Combine tomatoes, onion, beef and spices. Mix well. Place in meat loaf baking pan. Bake for approximately 1 hour at 350 degrees, brushing on liquid from pan as it is cooking.

Serves four   Total calories per serving: **265***
*Calorie content with bread crumbs **295**

SAUTÉED VEGETABLES ORIENTAL

	Calories
1 10 ounce box of favorite frozen vegetables	75
1 tbsp. safflower oil	120
⅛ tsp. light soy sauce	10
2 dashes of garlic powder	

Spray Silverstone frying pan with non-stick cooking spray. Place over low to medium flame. Pour in oil, soy sauce and sprinkle garlic powder. Spread this evenly around pan while heating. Add vegetables and separate with fork as much as possible. Cover and cook for 5–10 minutes, stirring occasionally. Serve as a side dish with meat or fish. Four ounces of any cooked meat—chicken, turkey or beef—can also be added directly to vegetables as they cook for a complete meal. Or serve this dish as a hungry-time snack.

Serves three   Calories per serving: **70**

THIN KIDS PIZZA

	Calories
½ English muffin, bagel or pocket pita	85
¼ cup of tomato sauce	25
Dash of oregano	
2 oz. mozzarella cheese	210
Sautéed vegetables or fresh mushrooms (optional)	

Layer sauce, optional vegetables and mozzarella cheese. Sprinkle on dash of oregano. Bake 15 minutes at 375 degrees or until cheese is golden brown.
Serves one   Total calories: **320**

CHICKEN PARMESAN

	Calories
4 ounces chicken cutlets	200
½ cup tomato sauce	50
1 ounce mozzarella cheese	100
Dash of oregano	

Bake chicken cutlets for 25 to 30 minutes at 325 degrees. Remove cutlets from oven and drain off any excess liquid. Add tomato sauce and oregano. Cover with mozzarella cheese. Bake for 30 minutes at 350 degrees.
Serves one   Calories per serving: **350**

CHICKEN IN THE POT

	Calories
1½ cups chicken soup*	75
4 oz. chicken cubes	200
½ cup fine egg noodles, cooked	100
Soup greens (including carrots)	10

Combine all ingredients in a large saucepan. Simmer over low heat until meat is cooked and vegetables are tender.
Serves one   Calories per serving: **385**

*See chicken soup recipe, p. 188

RECIPES

STRING BEANS ITALIAN CASSEROLE

	Calories
½ cup French-style string beans, cooked	25
½ cup cottage cheese or ½ cup ricotta cheese	120
½ cup low calorie tomato sauce	50
2 ounces mozzarella cheese	210
⅛ tsp. oregano	

Combine string beans, ricotta or cottage cheese, tomato sauce and oregano. Place in baking tin sprayed with non-stick cooking spray. Top with mozzarella cheese. Bake for 30 minutes at 405 degrees.

Serves one   Calories per serving: **405**

THIN KIDS FISH DELIGHT

	Calories
4 oz. fish filet (flounder, sole)	230
1 tbsp. light margarine	50
¼ cup lemon juice	5
1 tbsp. bread crumbs	30
⅛ tsp. paprika	
Dash of garlic powder	
Dash of black pepper	

In saucepan, melt margarine, combine and add lemon juice, paprika, garlic powder, and black pepper. Place fish in tin broiling pan. Cover fish evenly with margarine sauce. Broil until golden brown. Then bake fish at 350 degrees so that total cooking time (broiling and baking) is 20 minutes.

Serves one   Total calories: **315**

ORANGE CHICKEN SURPRISE

	Calories
6 ounces chicken (filet or parts)	200
4 tbsp. orange juice concentrate	50

Wash chicken and place on broiling tin. Brush orange juice concentrate over chicken. Bake for approximately 1 hour at 350 degrees or until chicken is tender when pierced with fork.

Serves one   Calories per serving: Approx. **250**

DRESSINGS AND SAUCE

YOGURT DIP DRESSING

	Calories
1 cup plain yogurt	150
3 tbsp. fresh or reconstituted lemon juice	10
⅛ tsp. mustard	
Seasoning to taste	

Combine ingredients in mixing bowl and blend thoroughly. Store in refrigerator and use as needed.

Yield: one cup   Calories per cup: **165**

BARBECUE SAUCE

	Calories
¼ cup tomatoes, pureed	25
½ cup water	
2 tsp. fresh or reconstituted lemon juice	3
1 tsp. dry mustard	3
1 tsp. Worcestershire sauce	14
1 tsp. chili powder	
½ tsp. garlic powder	

Blend ingredients and simmer over low flame for 15 to 20 minutes.

Yield: ½ cup   Calories per serving: **45**

OO-LA-LA FRENCHETTE DRESSING

	Calories
6 tbsp. salad oil	720
2 tbsp. red vinegar	5
⅛ tsp. pepper	
¼ tsp. dry mustard	

Combine all ingredients in a bowl or salad dressing bottle. Blend well.

Serves 7   Calories per serving: (approx.) **100**

RECIPES

DESSERTS

BAKED APPLE SWEETNESS
                                                                              Calories

   1 medium apple   65
   2 ounces apple juice   20

Wash and core apple. Place in small baking dish and cover with apple juice. Bake for approximately 30 minutes at 325 degrees or until apple is tender.
Serves one   Total calories: **85**

APPLE SURPRISE
                                                                              Calories

   1 lb. unpeeled apples   210
   ⅛ tsp. cinnamon
   ¼ cup whole raisins   120

Peel and chop apples. Mix with cinnamon and raisins. Smooth into pre-sprayed (or non-stick) pie tin. Bake for 30 minutes at 325 degrees. Great alone or as an addition to cottage cheese, plain yogurt, or hot cereal.
Serves three   Calories per serving: **110**

THIN KIDS ICE POPS
                                                         Calories

   6 oz. orange juice   90
   6 oz. pineapple juice   100
   6 oz. grape juice   120

Using any of the above unsweetened fruit juices, pour one into ice-pop makers, an ice-cube tray or paper cups. If using ice-cube tray or paper cups, cover tightly with plastic wrap and use toothpicks as handles. Freeze for at least 2 hours.
                                      Calories per serving: **90–120**

SNACKS

FROZEN GRAPE SENSATION   Calories
    20 seedless grapes   50

Remove grapes from stem and wash. Place in plastic bag or freezer container. Freeze for 1 to 2 hours.
Serves one   Total calories: **50**

FROZEN ORANGE SMILES   Calories
    1 medium navel orange   70

Peel orange and separate sections. Place in plastic bag or freezer container. Freeze for 1½ hours.
Serves one   Total calories: **70**

THE STICKS   Calories
    2 tbsp. peanut butter   210
    Celery pieces or apple slices   15–65

Spread peanut butter on apples or in grooves of celery.
Serves one   Total calories: **225–275**

FROZEN BANANA TREAT   Calories
    1 small banana   80

Peel banana and wrap banana in plastic wrap. Freeze for 1 to 2 hours.

Serves one   Total calories: **80**

CHAPTER XIV

FAT FREE FOREVER

Congratulations to you and to your child for working together and going through The Thin Kid Program as described in this book. You both have greatly contributed to your child's future health and well being. The path you have taken may not have always been easy, but the rewards, as you now can see, can last a lifetime.

You and your child have shared a close experience but there is still work ahead. Your challenge is just beginning. Some children assume that once they have lost the weight, they can go back to their old eating habits. It is *not* healthy for anyone of any age to lose and regain weight like a yo-yo. Therefore, the same careful approach we gave in this book for losing weight is the basic approach to maintaining slimness.

Children do have an advantage over adults. They grow and even if they gain a few pounds, they may still remain slim. They are also normally more active than adults, so that they do burn up more calories.

Remember that exercise, however, is a vital part of the program. With luck your youngster will find exercise tasks or some sport he likes enough to continue without urging. Your child will appreciate the toned muscles and sleek look of a well-exercised body.

When your child reaches or gets near goal weight—as specified by a physician—you should start increasing food from the four groups, one at a time, for a few days each. If you see no weight gain on the scales, then continue. For example, your child may be looking for more fruits or milk, so you could add another daily serving of each in two weeks until a level weight is maintained.

However, if your child begins eating high calorie foods again, weight will probably start to come back. Therefore, after you have invested all this time and energy and seen the thrilled look on your child's face after each weekly weigh in, focus on that rather than the foods to be added. If you see your child's weight going up too rapidly—and you should consult a physician on this—cut back on the foods, streamlining the original plan described in this book.

In some rare cases a child may lose weight too rapidly. If you or your physician believes this to be so, then, of course, add foods from the four food groups. We know that your child can take off weight safely and keep it off safely. The results, we are sure, will be rewarding to both you and your child.

We would like to hear your child's success story. You can write to us at 2165 Morris Avenue, Union, New Jersey 07083.

APPENDIX

FOOD GROUPS

Fruit Group *(Choose 3 daily.)*
1 medium fresh fruit (apple, orange, pear, 4 oz. plum)
1 oz. raisins
20 grapes or cherries
2 prunes or dates
1 small banana
⅛ honeydew melon
1 4 inch x 6 inch wedge of watermelon
½ cantaloupe
½ grapefruit
1 cup blackberries, blueberries, boysenberries, raspberries, or strawberries
½ cup fresh fruit salad
½ cup canned fruit, juice-packed
6 oz. unsweetened fruit juice
½ cup fresh pineapple chunks, unsweetened applesauce

Meat Group *(Choose 1 oz. serving for breakfast; 3 oz. serving for lunch, and 4 oz. serving for dinner.)*
Broil, boil, bake, or poach meat. Weigh meat after cooking. Eliminate gravy; trim off all fat. Remove skin from poultry after cooking. Each serving is equal to 1 oz. hard cheese, such as American or Muenster: Cooked lean beef, lamb, veal, pork, poultry, fish
¼ cup tuna or salmon
½ cup low calorie cottage cheese
1 tbsp. peanut butter
1 egg (limit to 3-4 eggs per week)

Milk Group *(Choose 3 daily.)*
1 cup skimmed or low fat milk
1 cup plain or low calorie yogurt

Treats *(Up to 3 times per week.)*
1 yogurt pop (uncoated)
1 low calorie ice-cream bar
½ cup low calorie ice cream

Fat Group *(Choose 3 daily.)*
1 tsp. butter, margarine, oil, mayonnaise or regular salad dressing
2 tbsp. diet salad dressing
1 tbsp. light margarine, light mayonnaise, sour cream, or cream cheese

Bread Group *(choose 2 to 3 daily.)*
½ English muffin
hot dog or hamburger bun
½ bagel
1 slice bread
2 Melba thin breads
1 pocket pita
2 rice cakes
5 Melba toasts
2 graham crackers
Any crackers to equal a 90-calorie serving
½ cup hot cereal
⅔ cup unsweetened cold cereal
1½ cups puffed wheat, etc.
¼ cup bread crumbs
½ cup pasta
½ cup rice
½ cup peas
½ cup corn
3 cups popcorn (air popped)
½ cup legumes
1 medium baked or boiled potato

Anytime Foods *(unlimited)*
Clear broth, water, seltzer, herbs, spices, seasonings, mustard, vinegar, horseradish, lemons or limes. Fresh-made vegetable juices and any vegetable except peas and corn.

Anytime Foods *(limited)*
8 oz. canned tomato or canned vegetable juice, ¼ tsp. table salt, 1 tsp. soy sauce, tsp. steak sauce, 1 tbsp. catsup, and ½ cup tomato sauce.